Praise for *Maiden to Mother*

"Sarah provides deep wisdom and guides us along the most important journey of our lives, from maiden to mother. This book is exactly what the feminine in each and every one of us needs in order to fully step into our fullest expression and our greatest power."

LeAnn Rimes
internationally acclaimed singer, songwriter,
and Grammy® Award winner

"I remember when I was at home giving birth to my first child, Brave. I had just begun active labor. I started to panic and call for my mother, Davi. My midwife came close and said, 'You are the mother now.' It was a powerful moment, an awakening. I was forced to let go of my maiden, ready or not. So many of us are thrust into Mother with nary a blueprint to guide us. Unmothered ourselves, this can be treacherous terrain. Sarah brings her gentle and deep wisdom to walk us through the ancient rites lost to us. Her words have helped me, and now they will help you."

Cree Summer
actress and singer

"*Maiden to Mother* is a timely and powerful book for all women to read and engage with. This time in history is what I call the 'Sophia Century'—a century that will be defined by the rising, maturing, and full self-expression of the feminine in women and also in men. Read this book, engage with the beautiful ideas in this book, and then find your wings and SOAR!"

Lynne Twist
bestselling author of *The Soul of Money*

"The words and teachings that Sarah shares so generously with the world are forged in the fire and heat of her fully lived experience. Vital and vulnerable, strong and tender, Sarah is a mystic, a wise woman, and a way-shower, and she will take you on an initiatory journey to deeply meet yourself, to navigate the terrain of womanhood, and to claim your power and presence. I hold Sarah in the deepest reverence. She, and all that she shares in the world, is fierce, much-needed medicine for us all."

Lisa Lister
bestselling author of *Witch* and *Code Red*

"At the heart of Sarah's book and work is a returning to ourselves in a society that has, in so many ways, attempted to pull us away from our essence. The work of *Maiden to Mother* invites us to remember, return to, and reawaken who we are underneath the conditioning we've received, in order to show up more fully, vibrantly, and wholly in our lives and within ourselves. This book is a balm, a gift, a mystical weaving of wisdom, and a nurturing companion that will ignite healing for so many."

Lisa Olivera
author of *Already Enough*

"Only Sarah Durham Wilson could make this tale so moving, so funny, so open, and so soulful, in words that sparkle like a love song. In *Maiden to Mother*, she goes intimately deep into grief, heartbreak, and spiritual rebirth. It's a bravely personal but universal guide to exploring the dark places of the heart and finding fresh wisdom there."

Rob Sheffield
contributing editor at *Rolling Stone* and
New York Times bestselling author

"Sarah Durham Wilson is giving voice and vocabulary to a swelling movement of people who want to cast off the inheritance of patriarchy but haven't seen a clear alternative. Reclaiming the feminine in all of her phases is the vital work Durham Wilson is engaged in, and I am thrilled that she's chosen to share it with us."

Caterina Scorsone
actress

"In a world that worships the maiden, this beautiful book is an invitation to move into the archetype of Mother, which is the most profound gift we can offer ourselves, our inner child, the earth, and the collective."

Ruthie Lindsey
speaker and author of *There I Am: The Journey from Hopelessness to Healing*

"*Maiden to Mother* is part archetypal medicine and part map for a woman's brave and loving return to a whole and healed self. Sarah Durham Wilson suffered a mother wound that nearly crushed her, and she has risen up and courageously found her way home to her own heart."

Sil Reynolds, RN
author of *Mothering and Daughtering: Keeping Your Bond Strong Through the Teen Years*

"Sarah Durham Wilson guides, teaches, and writes from an embodied place of having journeyed into the dark depths. Over the years of knowing her, I have seen this extraordinary witch enter deep communion with the Mother archetype, tending a most sacred relationship and thus feeding Her true force—so often forgotten by modernity. An offspring of her intimate soul journey is this book, and ultimately a contribution to the healing and resurrection of the Great Mother Goddess Creatrix energy so needed on our planet at these times. Sarah reminds us that it is by awakening, embodying, and living from the wholeness of the Mother archetype within us that the powerful love of Goddess will take her rightful place upon the living Earth."

Marysia Miernowska
author of *The Witch's Herbal Apothecary* and
director of The School for the Sacred Wild

Maiden
to
Mother

Sarah Durham Wilson

Maiden to Mother

Unlocking Our Archetypal
Journey into the Mature Feminine

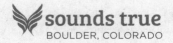
sounds true
BOULDER, COLORADO

Boulder, CO 80306

Published 2022

Cover design by Tara DeAngelis
Book design by Meredith March

The wood used to produce this book is from Forest Stewardship Council (FSC) certified forests, recycled materials, or controlled wood.

Printed in the United States of America

BK06086

Library of Congress Cataloging-in-Publication Data

Names: Durham Wilson, Sarah, author.
Title: Maiden to mother : unlocking our archetypal journey into the mature feminine / by Sarah Durham Wilson.
Description: Boulder, CO : Sounds True, 2022. | Includes bibliographical references.
Identifiers: LCCN 2021051067 (print) | LCCN 2021051068 (ebook) | ISBN 9781683647027 (hardback) | ISBN 9781683647034 (ebook)
Subjects: LCSH: Femininity. | Women--Identity. | Women--Psychology. | Self-actualization (Psychology)
Classification: LCC BF175.5.F45 D87 2022 (print) | LCC BF175.5.F45 (ebook) | DDC 155.3/33--dc23/eng/20211115
LC record available at https://lccn.loc.gov/2021051067
LC ebook record available at https://lccn.loc.gov/2021051068

10 9 8 7 6 5 4 3 2 1 (Impression)

To Avalon

Contents

Introduction

When you have no inner Mother,
Inside, you're still just a little girl
trapped in a woman's body.
Do you know that feeling?
I know it because I was her.
I was a little girl
Lost at sea
With no one
To watch over me.
Why don't I know how to live my life?
Why don't I have a map?
Why don't I have a key?

I thought I needed a map, but what I needed was a Mother—an inner Mother.

An idol of mine, the great Jungian analyst and author Marion Woodman, said if we don't tend to the fire inside, it will kill us. But if we nourish it, it will guide us.[1] She is referring to a voice inside that we often silence because it terrifies us: It will change everything we know. It will demand our greatness. It will require we accept the adventure life is calling us into. It calls us to the heroine's journey that we were born for.

So we ignore it, this voice of our destiny, of our ultimate destination. And ignoring that voice will bring us nothing but discontent. But if we can listen to this voice, accept its challenges, and expand instead of contract into suffering, we will find our true selves.

We must do this for ourselves—and the world—before it is too late. We must walk with beauty and courage. We must become the Mother: the Mother we needed when we were little and the Mother we need to be for ourselves now and for the world that is so desperately crying out for Mother. She is unconditionally loving, compassionate, wise, intuitive, infinitely creative, strong, sensual, serene, capable, fierce, gentle, reliable, a lover, and a queen.

Many women I work with initially think that our journey from Maiden to Mother must have something to do with their capacity to become mothers of children. After all, that is what the word *mother* means. Yet, I'm asking women to think about *mother* in an entirely new way. When I write about Mother, I'm referring to an archetypal mother, a birthright for all humans. This may or may not resonate with your experience of being mothered. It may also relate to your own experience of becoming the mother of a child, or it may not.

So many women can birth or raise children and remain in Maiden, which is the immature feminine. And, of course, we know so many women who age but don't mature. And unfortunately, what tends to happen when a woman is desperate to stay young on the outside is that she often stays young on the inside. And that's where it gets unnatural; that's where a woman becomes a wounded Maiden. Because to come into archetypal Mother is to come into the mature, fully developed, self-actualized feminine.

Introduction

When I say it is time to become the Mother, I mean:

It is time to do what you came here to do.
It is time to become who you came here to be.
I did this for myself before it was too late.
I want you to do this for your-
self before it is too late.
And I want you to do this for the
world before it is too late.

I sincerely believe the pain and losses we experience in wounded Maiden can be and are meant to be culled into the extraordinary wisdom of the Mother. That if we are willing, our pain will not be in vain. We can make meaning of our maiden pain, and we can turn it into Mother medicine. But first, we must face that pain. We must hear, tend to, and mother our inner little one: our Maiden, who has been deeply wounded by living in this patriarchal nightmare that told her she was bad or wrong, too much or too little.

All of my wounded Maiden's pain was not in vain; it has transformed into wisdom.

In Mother, our hearts break with compassion for ourselves and the world. And when the heart breaks, it expands to hold all of life. We can now hold ourselves and the other. In Mother, we learn to live more deeply, sensually awakened, and connected to our bodies and the Earth.

Through this journey, your pain won't be in vain either.

When I began Maiden-to-Mother work, I studied the behavioral blocks of my wounded Maiden state. My chief wound was not receiving the love of my mother as I desired it. She had never provided me with the security and acceptance that I craved, and before I knew it, she was gone. She died of cancer when I was seventeen, and we never had the chance in this life to reconcile and build a healthy connection. As a result, I developed the widespread feminine wounds of smallness, terror, hysteria, fragility, reactivity, vanity, and victimhood. I was desperate for attention and validation, and this was expressed in multiple abusive relationships with men.

In my early adulthood, I started developing a theory about this cultural paradigm in which women are abused, our desires and needs are suppressed, and our full power is never realized. This is a society in which toxic patriarchal masculinity grooms us to stay terrified little girls who serve men and appease conflict and never build the confidence to listen to our inner wisdom. Cultural messaging trains us to feel shame for being a woman who bleeds with the moon. We fear aging and believe that we are only as good as we look to the male eye through the patriarchal lens. The world's dominant religions reinforce that females are contaminating forces to the purity of the male and, therefore, must suppress their power. Potent conditioning descends on women, making us conform to this idea that we are secondary and less than our male counterparts. In America, this indoctrination begins early, when we read and are shown versions of Grimms' fairy tales that teach us that women are weak and need to be rescued by a handsome prince. The theme of such tales is woven into our popular culture and fed back to us as we mature, in the form of TV sitcoms, celebrity magazines, Hollywood romance movies, and subtle messaging in advertising. As a result, many women remain focused on the trivial and superficial aspects of femininity instead of understanding that the feminine is one of the most powerful, transformative forces in the universe.

Introduction

Do you feel stuck in girlhood, perhaps waiting for a prince and unable to progress into the power and confidence of a woman? If you do, it is not your fault. But it is your responsibility to examine the forces and circumstances that have arrested your development into the mature feminine. It is your duty to rewrite your fairy tale.

I was greatly influenced by the work of Marion Woodman, who at the time of her death in 2018 was heralded as the most influential explorer of the feminine psyche. The first half of her life was spent as an English and drama teacher, but in her forties, the prime time of feminine maturity, she discovered the psychological theories of Carl Jung and trained to become a psychoanalyst herself. She found that Jung's theories didn't necessarily apply to the female experience, as they were steeped in "patriarchal thinking." Her mission was to unearth previously hidden elements of the feminine unconscious, which would assist both women and men in their quest to become psychologically whole, conquering depression, anxiety, eating disorders, and other ailments. She used myth and poetry to help her clients and readers integrate these unconscious, primal needs of the feminine. This book includes my poetic interpretations of the Maiden-to-Mother journey in short passages throughout the chapters in homage to her.

In addition to drawing upon Woodman's insights, I offer up the ancient Sumerian myth of the Goddess Inanna as an example of a strong feminine that counters our dominant culture's ideas of the weak feminine. I use the ancient Goddess culture archetypes of the stages of a woman's life that mirror the cycle of nature from birth to death to rebirth. These are not the stages of life governed by the institutions of civilization, like birthdays, school graduations, first jobs, homes, marriages, raising children, and retiring. The transitions I present here are the biological ones accompanied by psychological shifts of increasing maturity reflected in the role a woman plays in relation to herself and others.

The Maiden archetype, like spring, like the waxing moon, is the healthy beginning phase of a woman's life—but it becomes unhealthy when we stay trapped in it, not progressing, not changing, never developing into the mature feminine. Like stagnant water, we get stuck somewhere on our path. And we stay in these small patterns of girlhood even though we are now in women's bodies.

In wounded Maiden, we have the great potential to develop into the mature feminine. Yet, to miss the full moon of our life, miss the Mother phase, miss our summer in full bloom is to miss our true life. That is the great tragedy of the modern feminine.

This stagnation occurs because the bridge we once crossed as women together, this Maiden-to-Mother rite of passage, has been erased. The bridge into our prime, into our power, has vanished. It has been buried in the dominant masculine energy that's currently pervasive in our culture, where men hold most positions of power, enjoy economic and political advantages over women, and still commit crimes against women that go unpunished every day. Despite decades of progress, our culture is still structured for the benefit of men and the subjugation of women. It is patriarchy.

There were many societies, cultures, and vast periods before the patriarchy intentionally targeted, quieted, and all but erased feminine power and matriarchal traditions worldwide. Women once gathered to be seen by each other and the Great Goddess, as we moved through the seasons of our lives, to witness and to honor our transformations into more mature roles. Around five thousand years ago, peaceful feminine-power worshipping cultures of the Near East were conquered by chariot-driving, sword-bearing warrior Indo-Europeans. These dominators ushered in a new era of male authority over women, secured by new modes of mass violence. Their patriarchal religion slowly demonized the figures of goddesses, a slow death that was capped by the fall of the Roman Empire. After that, the Christian church worked diligently to root out all traces of the old Goddess culture and the ideas of divine feminine power in order to assert the primacy of a male god. Today, we live with this legacy of the desecration of the female spirit. Women around the globe suffer horrific violence and live with vast inequality compared to the previous, more egalitarian era.

We all lost when we lost the Great Mother and when the Goddess—the feminine energy of God, woman as Creatrix, and the Great Mother of all—was vilified. When her covens, her temples, herstories, and the way of the feminine were destroyed and driven underground, we lost the village, we lost rituals, we lost each other, and we lost ourselves. I often ask, What would the world look like today if we still came together in community for rites of passage ceremonies oriented by the Goddess? The answer that I've come to is that when we rebuild the bridge from girl to woman, we can regain the power of the divine feminine.

Without rituals to mark milestones in our lives, we stagnate. In a rite of passage from Maiden to Mother, we would have laid down our wounded Maiden behaviors in offering as we crossed over into Mother—into the summer of our lives. With a deep need for that lost passage into Mother, I dug. Deep. And eventually, I found this transition we've been missing. I pieced it back together over years of trial and error and fire and failure until it was real, until I became real. I, a Motherless Maiden, grew up. I evolved into the mature feminine, as Marion Woodman termed it. I came into my power; I let my wise woman rise. I became safe for myself and safe for others, and I wrote it all down and turned it into a sort of Mother Map, a path from Maiden to Mother.

This Mother work has given my wounded Maiden the protective wise guidance she never had during those "train wreck" years. It's given her the voice of love and wisdom within that she never had in all her seeking. It saved her life. I learned how to walk with grace and strength, care for myself, tend to my wounded Maiden, live my soul life, and offer my soul gift. I've helped hundreds of women across this bridge, from girl to woman. Now, if you're here, it's your time, too.

On behalf of our feminine collective, I am so grateful you're here.

I need to begin by stating that I know this book is flawed because I come from a singular perspective—that of a cisgendered, heterosexual white woman of European origin who was privileged to grow up with financial security and good health. I'm now a single mother of a precious daughter who enjoys the support of a wide community of people seeking the wisdom of the divine feminine. I work with groups of women, holding space for their transformation at retreats several times a year. I also work with individual clients on their Maiden-to-Mother journeys. I hope that this book contains universal elements that will support all of your identities, whether you're queer, non-binary, BIPOC, from a marginalized or targeted group, rich, poor, differently bodied, or neurodivergent. Whatever wonderful traits make up the authentic you, this book shows you a different path from the dominant narrative of our culture.

This book is an initiation, which means entering a portal to a new way of life. The first thing you need to do is say yes to this journey. You're going to have to find a quiet place in your life, right now in this bookstore or standing in the kitchen, whether you're in the fetal position or strong-spined, wherever you are, however you are, is welcome. You're just going to close your eyes and enter your inner world where your Mother lives and know that the Goddess is listening to you.

This will not be an overnight transition. The Goddess works with you deeply and slowly, and mysteriously. But you'll know it has been real because, by the end of this journey, you'll have been forged into womanhood by fire, better able to embody Mother and tend your wounded Maiden until she becomes the healthy Maiden. This Maiden will never leave you—she is an inner rebelle creative genius—free to rest and play and dream and be seen for her gifts.

You're going to have to say, "Yes. Yes, I'm ready to be the Mother."

In doing this, you're saying yes to the end of one way of life. Yes to the death of your smallness, your helplessness. Your self-sabotage. Your reactivity. Your wait to be saved.

Now you're at one end of a bridge—the end of your Maiden life—and you're going to have to walk across this bridge.

Are you ready?

Growing Out of Maiden

To my unMothered women,
To my survivors,
And my wounded Maidens,
There was never anything wrong with you
There was something wrong with them.

My adult life followed a predictable script: I'd hop into one car of a fantastic opportunity, take it up to one hundred miles an hour—probably drunk—crash it, and walk away. I'd leave it burning on the side of the road, a mess for someone else to clean up. Then, I'd jump into a new car glimmering with a new opportunity, and I'd retake the wheel, definitely drunk, stoned, or sedated; accelerate to a hundred miles an hour; crash; and leave it burning on the side of the road. Race, crash, repeat.

Then, one day, I ran out of chances. I ran out of bridges to burn.

It turns out that was a brutal gift.

I'd had several moments when I knew I could change the pattern, and I would succeed for a time. One of these powerful realizations came, not dramatically at the edge of a cliff overlooking sea-bashed cliffs or while meditating on mushrooms, but in a mundane moment as I stood in line at the grocery store.

It was March on Martha's Vineyard, the island off the coast of New England where I lived, and the sky was like an unappetizing gray, foggy soup. It is the time of year that feels bleak rather than idyllic when you yearn for the bursting forth of flowers or the orgasmic blasts of green that you know will be arriving soon but have not yet come. During these last long days of winter, I spent periods wondering if I was alive, or perhaps if I was already in the afterlife and trapped in limbo, not yet assigned to heaven or hell. I felt like a ghost.

I was raising a nine-month-old baby on my own, and I lived in a shabby rented apartment above a garage. The neighbors next door were dealing heroin, and there was no end to the trouble they were causing at odd hours in the night.

To all outward appearances, my life was not going so well.

It may have looked as if I had given up. I had indeed fallen to the bottom.

I held my doula's hand during my C-section, and afterward, my father visited me for a short time. I remember savoring every single moment, wishing it would last, and asking the night nurse to tell me her life story so she'd stay by my side. From then on, though, my baby daughter and I were mostly alone, first in the hospital and then at home. It was a bleak time in my life. It was all I could do just to complete the bare minimum of keeping us both alive. I merely survived. The idea of thriving didn't occur to me, as it would have seemed as ambitious as landing on the moon, and I barely ever left my house. The idea of a supportive community—or a village—was the furthest from my mind, but it was what I most needed.

I was in the underworld, which I had visited several times before. I was feeling all the darkness. Yet, at the same time, I was brewing a potion for my healing.

I know it is possible to choose to resign ourselves to the underworld. I heard the Jungian analyst Marie-Louise von Franz characterize this as: "Every dark thing one falls into can be called an initiation. To be initiated into a thing means to go into it. The shamans say that becoming a medicine (wo)man begins by falling into the power of the demons. The one who pulls out of the dark place becomes the medicine (wo)man. And the one who stays in it is the sick person."

I was in the transition zone where we choose to stay dark and sick or we choose to get well and rise in the light.

At times like this in the past, I would cast and read runes. My mother had a set of stones inscribed with potent symbols, used by Nordic and Germanic tribal cultures across northern Europe, Scandinavia, and Britain for literary, divination, and magical purposes. Runes are a kind of oracle, like tarot cards, that are useful for hinting at answers to your spiritual questions when you have limited information. They don't predict the future, however. You must use your intuition to figure out the insight they cull from your subconscious.

My mother never shared anything about her runes; I just learned about them from playing with them as a child. The stones and symbols just made sense to me. A long time after she died, I found a box in the basement containing more runes, spell books, and tarot cards that she must have consulted. This was her hidden feminine power that I can only imagine she was somewhat ashamed of. For me, discovering and learning more about using these tools of intuition helped me uncover my divine feminine.

So I cast runes. I was drawn to the power of the Isa stone, which counsels that we must watch for signs of spring; in the underworld, however, we can become blind to them or even give up on them ever appearing again. If you're lucky like I was, something or someone lights a stick of dynamite underneath you, and you get blown out of the darkness. But so many women remain asleep as if under a curse, waiting in the casket for the prince to kiss them awake. They've forgotten their power and that they've got to rise and fight.

Women can awaken from the curse of a system that would prefer for the feminine to stay "under the world"—and not in it—forever. This is the lava-exploding-from-the-dormant-volcano moment. This was the intersection where I stood and where I wallowed—temporarily, for I had the power of the Isa rune.

I was in line at the grocery store, utterly resigned to my new lifeless normal, standing under aggressively bright fluorescent lights with my baby sleeping in her carrier on my chest. I realized —once again—that I didn't have enough money to buy the few groceries that rolled down the conveyor belt. When the toll reached $45, the blood had drained from my face, and my hands were shaking. I knew I only had $32 left in my account.

I looked meekly into the eyes of the clerk.

"I'm sorry," I squeaked. "I have to put some things back."

She nodded.

"It's tough having a baby on your own," she says. "I know. I did it too."

I could feel the man behind me stiffen. This was uncomfortable for *him*. He stared at his shoes.

"Excuse me," I said, turning toward him on my way to return the armful of food I couldn't afford. But the woman behind the register kindly saved me.

"You can just leave what you can't pay for here," she said.

Minutes later, the small bundle of groceries I could afford sat in the old beach car I'd borrowed from my father and his wife. I'd had to sell my own car to make rent. My phone rang. It was my aunt, someone I trusted and admired. I answered with a lonely waiver in my voice. I was desperate to connect.

"Your sister called me," she said. "She told me you borrowed money again."

"Yes—I—I have some ideas. I'm going to make it—I just need a little more time . . ."

"And she and I agreed," she interrupted. "It's time you go on welfare."

This was the strike of the match, and the drawing it down toward the dynamite's wick.

Then she said: "It was a good dream." She was referring to my desire to devote myself to women's writing and teaching. "I'm not saying you should give up on it. I'm saying you need to be realistic."

Yet this is what I heard: "We have given up on you, and we think you should too."

Ostensibly, what she said made sense. Everything in my life at that moment looked dark and depressing.

The call to rise from the lair of self despair and to become a heroine comes in many forms. Mine came as that phone call from my aunt on a wet, cold, gray morning in the grocery store parking lot, holding on to my napping baby, after being unable to purchase enough food.

I needed to make a choice—in that very moment.

Part of me wanted to give up and tell my aunt, "Yes, you're right." But my entire body convulsed at this idea.

You see, I had been working on something in the dark: I had been following a splinter-thin sliver of light out of my endless night. I was piecing together the puzzle of my life that needed deep time in the underworld to become whole.

With that phone call, for which I am endlessly grateful, I knew this was the time to bring my project into the light. Because if you're not careful, you'll become too careful. You'll lose your nerve. You'll never try again. You'll stay closed for life. The time to shine was upon me though. Life was presenting me with a choice: rise with my dream or stay in the underworld forever and never come back up. Rebirth is a risk. I chose to embrace this opportunity because, as a famous quote by Elizabeth Appell reads, "The day came when the risk to remain tight in a bud was more painful than the risk it took to blossom."[2]

That phone call lit the dynamite's fuse, and I exploded out of the underworld. It didn't matter if I was ready or not. I steeled myself and told my aunt: "I've got this." This moment would become a seminal Mother teaching. I stopped waiting or looking around for someone to make it alright. I declared it would be. My declaration willed it so. Knowing that I had my own back and that I would find a way to support my daughter, I finally felt free. I was free to create what would become a successful portal for women to embrace the Maiden-to-Mother journey. I used this experience to fuel my emerging business, and within a few months, I had no problem buying what I needed at the store. In fact, my work would go on to create savings. In this light, my work saved me.

There are women who stay in the underworld through no fault of their own: it is a byproduct of a male-dominated society. It goes like this: If women are not initiated into Mother through rites of passage, which are the tools of rebirth, they are unable to evolve. They age, but they never transform. They do not mature or self-actualize, so they remain infantilized and dependent.

The alternative is to decide to heal and claim maturity. We evolve and bloom on the inside, and the bloom manifests on the outside. That life force blesses everything in our wake.

The ground was falling out beneath my feet, and I was holding a child in my arms. Had I been alone, I might have let myself fall—but I would not let my baby girl fall. At a moment when I couldn't act for myself, I could act for something greater than myself.

The end phase of the Isa rune is when the ground of the upperworld is thawing, while the underworld is burbling with life, in a state of rearrangement. Spring had arrived, and I could not stop my body coming back to life, even if sleeping and hiding felt far more comfortable. I was moving into the realm of the Inguz rune: the rune of new beginnings, which tells us to shed our ruts and bad habits. It urges us to move beyond the deeply set patterns of behavior that only work with the selves we used to embody. Yet it also cautions that rebirth is a dangerous undertaking.

Still, I had to make a move.

You might want to turn around and head back to where you came from during the passage from Maiden to Mother. You might even want to curl up into the fetal position, suck on a bottle of Chardonnay, and give up. But Maureen Murdock, who wrote *The Heroine's Journey*, would call turning around and going back to your wounded Maiden wiring, aborting your process of rebirth. If you're here, truly on the threshold, you can't go back. By the time you're asking if you can just return to the familiar (but suffocating) way things were, it's too late—the bridge behind you has crumbled.

The passage is long, dangerous, and dark. Your Maiden is exhausted from a fearful, reactive, and terrifying life with no one to save her despite whatever she was promised in the fairy tales of a Goddess-less culture. Like in fairy tales we are all indoctrinated with as children, there will be dragons, but here the Maiden must fight for herself. But she is saving herself from beneath the glass, kissing herself alive instead of waiting for a Prince Charming with a hero complex to rescue her from the dragon.

As the poet Rilke wrote, "Perhaps all the dragons in our lives are princesses who are only waiting to see us act, just once, with beauty and courage. Perhaps everything that frightens us is, in its deepest essence, something helpless that wants our love."[3]

Beneath those terrifying and painful obstacles, those fire-breathing dragons on your passage, are your Maiden wounds that have been steering your ship into wrecks. These are almost always the same for each of us: a deep-rooted sense of unworthiness, a constant sense of danger, a lack of self-trust, and feeling loveless, abandoned, and that you are "bad."

The Mother in you must tend to those wounds and act with beauty and courage. Because while life happens to the Maiden, life happens through the Mother. The wounded Maiden can only try to survive in the waves; in calling on the Mother, we become the ocean.

The woman with an inner Mother braces herself. She closes her eyes. She breathes. She returns to the throne, the place of internal power. She roots down to the Mother Well, where all is deeply well. She asks for the strength and wisdom and power of the Great Mother Goddess. She doesn't react. She waits for the answer, and then she responds. She pulls up the faith inside of her like buried treasure from the Earth. Fear will flirt with her, asking: "But don't you want to freak out?"

The Mother pauses. "My wounded Maiden is tempted. But I've been here before. I know this place. Fear got me nowhere.

Faith moved me along. I was weak for too long. And now, it's time to be strong."

As I write this, above my desk, there are beautiful white roses that have erupted from their buds. They are in full bloom. They are one of my favorite metaphors for the Mother. These gorgeous blossoms became this powerful and this beautiful by reaching peak fulfillment and self-actualization after rooting deep into the earth, pushing up through great darkness, rising, risking, and blasting open their tiny, confined buds. And in their most receptive and vulnerable state, they are their most powerful. They are in their prime.

They are us.
They have to open to life
to live.
If you're ready to bloom, read
on. You're at the crossing.
What feelings or events have brought you here?
What initiated you to this crossroads?
Why are you here?
What kind of life do you have now?
What kind of life do you want?

I promise you the messages in this book will change your life if you claim them as your own. I promise that you'll become your own heroine. If you walk with me, you'll become a Mother to yourself.

You'll also become a Mother to the world.

We will bloom and come into our full moon together. We know that after the full moon comes the waning, after the

Mother becomes the Crone. After the bloom, our bodies return to the earth. Don't miss the full moon of your life. Let's bloom together by uncovering the buried ancient feminine.

Together we'll integrate our wounded Maiden traits back into the lap of the Great Mother. We will learn the practices of self-mothering. I'll share with you how to cross the bridge from Maiden into Mother, and I'll tell you about my initiation into this phase. We'll travel with Sumerian Goddess Inanna, who gave us the map to feminine rebirth. We'll follow her down through the underworld to meet her severed dark sister, Ereshkigal, who holds the key to our power.

And we'll rise again.

We'll learn how to meet and call on the Mother through practicing rituals and by strengthening our intuition. We will explore true internal beauty and restore the grace in becoming wise, older women. Many women have gone down this path before us, and we will also call on their guidance and wisdom to direct us as we proceed. We will offer compassion to ourselves at every step of the way, and we will alchemize our burdens into offerings. I invite you to experience this transformation at your own pace and in your own way.

As we walk the pages of this book together, this process will require you to spend time reflecting, integrating, and going inward. At the end of each chapter, I've included journaling prompts, meditations, and visualizations to support your process further.

A few things to keep in mind for these prompts:

1. What you put in is what you'll get out. If you're rushing through these pages, your immersion will only go so deep. This will not be an overnight transition. The Goddess works with you deeply, slowly, and mysteriously. Take your

time, grab some tea, find a quiet spot, and let the Goddess lead you each step of your journey.

2. As you reflect, do your best to trust your process. Let every exercise take you closer to your intuition and power. Avoid overthinking or overanalyzing. Go deeper than your head, allowing your body and soul to lead you.

3. It might be helpful to begin a new journal so you have all your Maiden-to-Mother resources in one place. Don't limit yourself to the reflection exercises I've offered here. Always keep writing if you feel inclined, letting the Great Mother guide the pen.

Let's start with our first exercise.

Reflection Exercise: Crossing the Threshold

Close your eyes and imagine a hand-built wooden bridge over a large river. The sun has just broken through the clouds, and you can feel the warmth on your skin. Imagine this bridge crossing will lead you to your destiny to become your own heroine and Mother. This path is sacred and available to you. Notice what you feel in your body and what it feels like to embark on a great inner journey.

This is the beginning of the passage to your new self.

As you gaze at the bridge, consider what you're most excited about and what you are apprehensive about. Trust your body to show you what is most vital for you to know as you prepare to cross over.

Take your first step by opening up your journal, and use the prompts below as you begin to write.

JOURNAL PROMPTS

What excites you most about crossing this threshold? What are you looking forward to? What do you desire most?

What fears or apprehensions do you have? Where do you feel them in your body? Begin practicing your self-mothering and place a hand on your body where you feel the fear. Is there anything your fear might need to dissolve? Courage? Strength? Love?

What brought you to the Maiden-to-Mother journey at this time? Did you have a moment like I did, running out of cash at the grocery store, that spurred you on?

What daily practices might you need to support your journey? Better nutrition? More movement? Other forms of self-care?

What dreams are whispering in your heart? What is your biggest dream for your life?

Now you're at one end of a bridge—the end of your Maiden Life—and you're going to have to walk across this bridge. So here we go . . .

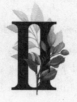

The Descent of Inanna

One day I looked in the mirror and asked,
"Oh no, where did my looks go?"
And a voice from deep within answered,
"They went down below
True beauty lives in a place far beneath your face
And to retrieve it,
It is down below
You must go."

In Monica Sjöö and Barbara Mor's feminist classic, *The Great Cosmic Mother*, the authors wrote about the stones of Avebury, the largest standing Neolithic circle of stones. The stones are located near the village of Avebury in southwest England and once served as monuments for the Goddess. They were a site for rituals, rites of passage, sacrifices, and celebrations. This was a place where humans practiced an earth-based religion that honored the seasons and the corresponding lifecycle stages of humanity.

"Here every year anew, the Goddess was born, grew into maiden and lover, became mother, and finally the old hag of death," wrote Sjöö and Mor. "The temples were her seasonal reality, and the people moved with her from place to place in rhythm with the changing farming year."[4]

Once upon a matriarchal time, women gathered in sacred council to witness and honor the preeminent passages of each other's lives.

Imagine visiting the stones of Avebury twenty-three hundred years ago and being ushered through your rite of passage into maturity, into your season of Mother. Women are gathered all around you inside the circle of towering stones, which seem to peer down at you as great elders. They are like wise, stone beings who have witnessed every woman walk through this portal before you.

Under the warm sun, you stand barefoot in the early summer grass; a white linen shift drapes over your body. Your hair is free and wild, like the wild woman you are. The village priestess beckons you forth. Your name is called loudly, echoed by the stones. The first act of your life, the youth, the Maiden, the springtime, is over. The curtain now closes on your Maiden phase.

The women in the circle, all the Mothers who have passed through this rite before you, close their eyes. Together you honor and hold vigil for your youth, your innocence, and for the lessons arising from your life's troughs and peaks, without which you could not have become wise. You honor your time of yearning, of searching and becoming, and then you release it, with love and gratitude.

The priestess asks you to step over a small threshold. It's woven with branches and moss and sits at the center of the stones. With this crossing, you step into Mother. You accept your maturity and your power. The seeking phase is over, your time of becoming is over, and you embrace your responsibility as Mother on the path to Crone. In Maiden, others were responsible. In Mother, you are. You are a mother to yourself and your community. You are a mother to the Earth, and you're becoming a future elder for the village.

You root your strong bare feet into the summer earth, raise your arms to the open sky bridging heaven and Earth with the vessel of your body, and you claim your powers of creation. At this moment, the Mother accepts her seasonal reality: the passing nature of life, the changing of seasons, aligned with Mother Earth. The Mothers of your community walk toward you and crown you with a garland of blossoms. You are Mother too. They welcome you into the summer of your life. The wind picks up, and the other women dance around you, and nature showers you with her blessing.

I once thought my rite of initiation out of maidenhood would be, as so many wounded Maidens believe, a wedding. This is what our culture has instilled in us as the moment of transformation from Maiden to Mother, in place of our original feminine rite of passage. The fairy tales we are marinated in since childhood usually end with the young maiden meeting her prince and marrying him.

In the fairy tale version of my life, my mother had died, and just like Cinderella or Snow White, my father chose a new wife. As these plot lines paralleled the childhood stories I had heard about orphaned heroines, so I believed that I, too, would live out the script, and a man would come to rescue me.

But one month before our wedding, my fiancé called it all off.

We had technically broken up, but because I'd begged for it, we were still spending a lot of time together, mourning what could have been. On one of our last days together, we went to see the movie *Julie and Julia*, written by one of my idols, Nora Ephron. She had a way of rendering her women characters so lovingly. They were messy and lost, but they had hope and they eventually found their way home to themselves. When the film ended, I was surprised to see that he had started to cry.

"What's the matter?" I asked. "I mean," I shrugged self-consciously, "besides everything?"

"You're wasting yourself. You could be like Nora Ephron, Sarah. You could. I know you, I know your writing. But you don't even try. It's terrible to watch someone so good at something not even do it. Or do anything, for that matter. What happened to you?"

I couldn't answer. I didn't know.

I did know I was all potential and no follow-through. After years of trying the writing life, I had not ended up where I thought I would.

My career had started when I interned at *Rolling Stone* magazine. From there, I went on to various roles at VH1, *GQ*, *Vanity Fair*, and when I met Tim, I was writing for *Interview* magazine. That was the successful veneer. Beneath the surface, I was terrified, scrambling, showing up late and hungover, sabotaging myself at every turn. Five years into my rock-n-roll journalist dream, it had become so hollow. Why was I not happy when I had achieved what I'd claimed as my dream? I know now that it was my deep wounded Maiden traits that kept me from maturing professionally. And my vulnerability as a woman seeking constant approval allowed some to take advantage of me and wound me.

After my internship at *Rolling Stone*, I interned at a popular indie music magazine. The editor was a brash British man named Charlie who never took me seriously. He'd either ignore me or flirt with me. One day he shouted a question over his back, and I was the only one who knew the answer. It was a question about the band that my future fiancé, a singer-songwriter, played in, and I was an encyclopedia on his specific indie rock scene.

Charlie turned around, impressed. "So, you're more than just a pretty face, huh?" From him, this was a high compliment, and I blushed. That night the staff went to a concert where, as usual, everyone got plastered. On the walk to the bar afterward, Charlie pushed me up against an alley wall and forced himself on me without my consent—yes, date rape.

I couldn't go back to work the following day; I was devastated and mortified. That afternoon, a female editor called me.

"I can't come back," I said. She was quiet. "Okay," she said. "I understand. I just want to know, was it Charlie?"

"Yes," I said.

She sighed.

"I'm sorry," she said, and hung up. In my twenties in New York, I would get used to date rape. And I would always tell myself I deserved it, that it was my fault, I was loose, I was wild, I was drunk, I was slutty, I was a groupie. But I know that I was desperate for male attention to fill the wounds that my self-love could have helped me heal.

I met Tim, the man I would be engaged to, in a dark East Village bar while on a date with another rock front man. I was in the habit of tossing back several drinks a night, quickly sliding into alcoholism. I couldn't stop, but I wanted someone to stop me, put their arms around me, and make me feel totally safe with them. I wanted them to Mother me. I wanted them to ask me if I was okay—because clearly, I wasn't. I regularly showed up hungover at work in the previous night's clothes, missed deadlines, and cried at my desk. Now I can recognize that I did this because I was so unMothered.

When we met, Tim slid in next to me in the wooden booth with a mischievous, sweet smile. Jokes and joy billowed up from his being, and we quickly became like bear cubs, laughing and playing along the streets of New York City. At one point that night, I just left my original date. Tim gently pushed me up against a wall to kiss me, and it felt like a vow written with our tongues. It was crazy, but we charted the rest of our lives together, our meeting was so potent that we were sure we were one another's forever, and I thought he would be all I ever needed. We fused like stars. I felt like my search for purpose was over. He was my dream come true.

As our relationship grew and he invited me to move to his hometown of Omaha, I saw the opportunity as a life raft from the ship of my life that was about to capsize. He was Orpheus, the god of music, and I was his tree-nymph lover, Eurydice. And when I landed in Nebraska, I stopped writing. Fueled by the morals of fairy tales, I thought I was a princess who a knight had saved, and I would never again have to fight. I could collapse in his arms and fall asleep.

But that willingness to surrender meant that I was stuck in my smallness like so many wounded Maidens. I was unused potential, I was asleep in my calcified bud—or that glass coffin you see the princesses in as they await their prince's kiss. I had been conditioned my whole life to think that once a man rescued me, I could just relax and stop my quest. But when I surrendered to that conditioning, I died even more inside. My depression, anxiety, and suicidal desires that started after my mother died came back to haunt me because I stopped using my gifts.

That year, on one of his records, Tim wrote a song called "What Have I Done?" about a man wasting his life with a woman who was wasting hers. In another song, I remember him howling about me, "How can you take what you cannot give?" I was always demanding more—more love and trust when I had none to offer in return. The less love and trust I had for myself, the more I grew like a hungry ghost for his. I would take it from him only to be starving again the next day. I took all his love and trust until he had none left. Without an inner source of my own love, I was endlessly starving for it from others. Inside I felt absolutely empty and atrophied.

He was right: I could take, but I could not give.

We tried to resuscitate my career by moving to Los Angeles, but I had become addicted to alcohol and Valium, and I thought seriously about killing myself. The substance use and even the longing for death were my attempt to seek the Mother's comfort—but I didn't know that then. I got jobs and promptly lost them, never finding my footing. Though it felt like death, our pre-wedding breakup saved my life. Like Orpheus did to Eurydice, Tim left me stranded in the underworld.

Years later, I would learn about an ancient Sumerian myth of a woman's time in the underworld. This story would inspire me, parallel my life more than any fairy tale, and give me the strength to actualize the heroine's power instead of waiting for a man/savior to complete my life.

Created some fifty-five hundred years ago, the myth of Inanna, the Sumerian Queen of Heaven and Earth, begins with her marriage to a handsome young shepherd. It should have been a time of grand celebration, but instead, she heard a dreadful cry from below.

The painful shriek was from her sister, Ereshkigal, who was lamenting the death of her husband. Inanna wished to go down to the underworld, where Ereshkigal lived, to attend the funeral rites and be with her sister in her mourning. As I understand it, Ereshkigal represents the dark, separated part of the divine feminine. Symbolically, Inanna wanted to sit with her own pain and confront her shadow by joining her sister below. She wanted to descend to the dark feminine and reclaim her wholeness.

But everyone around Inanna said, "No. No one ever returns from the underworld. If you go, you'll never come back."

Determined to follow the call and meet her destiny, Inanna went anyway, and told her faithful servant, Ninshubar: "If I don't come back in three days, call to the fathers for help."

At the entrance of the underworld, Ereshkigal's attendants barred its seven gates. "The rules of the underworld are perfect, and not to be questioned," they told her.

Ereshkigal ordered her servants to seize one of Inanna's worldly possessions at each of the seven gates. She would finally enter Ereshkigal's lair the way a tree meets the cold heart of winter, as her barest self. By the time she arrives at the underworld, Inanna has been stripped from crown to gown: she is naked and bowed low. In her grief, fury, and judgment, Ereshkigal strikes and kills Inanna, hanging her corpse on a meat hook.

Three days pass, and Inanna's servant Ninshubar begins to seek help. The first two kings refuse. They say Inanna has broken the rules by going to the underworld, and she must be punished. (This part of the myth is that cruel, but necessary, moment when a woman realizes that her god and government only protect the obedient.) It is only father God Enki, God of the feminine water element, who responds with a way to save Inanna. He carves two "galla," or small "demon flies," from the clay beneath his fingernails, gives them life, and sends them to the underworld, where they find Ereshkigal moaning on the floor. She is wailing in grief. "My husband is dead! I've killed my sister!" They compassionately listen and witness Ereshkigal's sorrow and pain, telling her the truth she needs to hear. "Your husband is dead. You've killed your sister." Their witnessing the moment causes Ereshkigal to soften, and she agrees to give Inanna's corpse to them. They feed it, and after a while, Inanna comes back to life. And she comes back self-actualized. She has faced death to know life, and she has reclaimed her shadow. She is whole. This is the key to our healing: by hearing herself, she heals herself.

The story of Inanna is universal, and nearly every one of my students works with it as a parable of her own life. It's also timeless because although it was written in antiquity, it represents the eternal plight of a woman at a crossroads: to continue to follow the crowd or to follow her own soul. Through this trial, she learns to follow what she thinks and trust what she feels.

Imagine that you are Inanna, Queen of Heaven and Earth, living in modern times. You know the upper realms quite well, too well. You're far too comfortable on autopilot. You have been surviving in—but never thriving in—the patriarchy.

On the outside, everything is fine. The fathers have approved of you, the good girl. You have done everything you've been told to do. You've lived for everyone else's approval. You've done everything right, maybe you've gotten married, perhaps you've succeeded at your job or motherhood, and people like you. But you are still not whole; you've still got a gaping hole inside you. Something is desperately missing—and it's you.

Soon, you start to hear a call from deep inside. In an exhausted sense of surrender, you know that the answers you need will not come from outside of you. You know that because you've looked everywhere else, except inside of you. You've spent your life learning from other people, through schools and programs, online courses, books, teachers, and trainings. Nothing has stuck but you. You're at the threshold between Maiden (a child to whom things happen) and Mother (an adult, whom things happen through).

Nothing you've found outside of yourself has sustained true peace and fulfillment within. Maybe others' wisdom, guidance, or advice held you up for a minute, but its sturdiness was as sustainable as a wobbly post, and you've fallen back to the ground. You keep being led back here. Back to the Earth. Back to your body. Back to you and the door you've been distracted from opening your whole life. Finally, no doors are left but the one that leads inside of you. This is the cave of you, which, as the great Joseph Campbell so famously said, "leads to the treasure you seek."[5]

This is the thing about treasure: it's buried. You don't find it on a sunny day walking through the park, tripping over it as you skip through bliss. You only find it in the dark when you face your greatest fears. To continue looking outside of yourself is an endless, fruitless trap. The current consumerist, capitalistic culture would be very happy if you kept trying to find yourself in external validation. Do not feed the culture. Instead, feed the life source of your soul.

Stop the running, chasing, and reaching for the summit of the infinite mountain that leads to nowhere. Slip off your shoes and press your bare feet deep into the earth. Leave the race to nowhere. Get still by the river of your life. Just stop. Drop your expectations. Just watch. Just look. Just breathe. Where are you trying to go? Who are you trying to be? Has the way you've been walking gotten you any closer to what you're trying to attain? Is doing actually the way to your desires? Or is "simply being" the real answer that feeds your soul?

All of our combined lust for bigger, better, and more has created the harm we've done to ourselves, others, and the Earth. We have become lost in a labyrinth outside of ourselves, but the key to our self-realization is already hanging from our neck.

This is the gift that comes from being stopped in your tracks and being pulled into the underworld: you cannot take another step in a life that is not yours. You can't go any farther down the wrong road. A dark grace has arrested your progress and made you face your soul's longing over your mind's programming. You must stop now, before it's too late and you lose your life to others' commands and demands.

Because you couldn't stop yourself, the Goddess has stopped you, here at this crossroads. You have a choice: to go the way you've always gone, in the world you've always lived in, or to dream up and create a new world. Take the key from around your neck and open the door to Mother.

Her world is one of immeasurable inner treasure. The Mother has stopped filling the hole in her soul with lifeless crap and meaningless relationships. She will empty it to fill it with her creations. She wants less, not more. A woman at this transition into truth finds she is moving through a portal, like the trees in winter, like a child from the womb to the world. She can only take herself. Nearly everything but the soul must be shed to pass into archetypal Mother. Houses, jobs, relationships, and not least, her ways of thought that stem from patriarchal consciousness cannot come with her. This is the death of one form of consciousness that allows us to birth another.

Because we do not, as a culture, practice rites of passage outside of institutional progressions, there is no invitation to honor life or to mature. Not only are we not aligned with our seasonal realities of a life's spring, summer, fall, and winter, we are the opposite—we live in ignorance and fantasy of a false stability. We live as if we will not die, and in turn, as if the Earth is indestructible as well.

Our culture will exhaust you, or has already. It will commodify you, objectify you, erase your humanity, and keep you waiting for a magic prince. It will be a race you never win. It will kill you early. It will steal your soul. It will leave you feeling dejected, bitter, resentful, and remorseful at the end of your "life," as if you hadn't really lived at all. Because you hadn't. Maybe for others, but not for yourself. And that is no way to live. So leave the race, and leave it now.

Dissent, and descend.
She had to go to hell
To find out who the hell
She really was
And just like Inanna
She came back
A Hell of a Woman

Reflection Exercise:
A Review of Inanna's Descent

In the story of Inanna, the Sumerian
Goddess has just married a handsome
shepherd and appears to "have it all together."
Then she hears a deep calling within that
changes her life forever. This is her dark
Goddess sister, Ereshkigal, who is not a
biological sister as it may appear in the story,
but rather a part of her soul that is crying
out. Ereshkigal is all the forsaken parts of
Inanna that call her to go deeper to discover
her true self. Inanna cannot deny the
magnetic force to descend to the underworld
to reclaim the buried and severed parts of
herself. She does not know what is in store
for her just yet; she only knows she cannot
deny this calling and must go at any cost.

EXERCISE 1:

Spend some time allowing the story of
Inanna to enter and saturate you. Take a
few deep breaths, feeling the chair in which
you're sitting, and really get into your body,
leaving the outer world behind.

Think of all the ways in the past that you've looked outside of yourself for answers, guidance, and approval. Now go inward and pay attention to the truth of you—your soul—begging for your attention. Those parts of you that you were told were bad or wrong or weird, those parts of you that can only be reclaimed in the darkness, are the inner voice calling to you now, just the way Ereshkigal called out to Inanna. After all, you keep being led back here, don't you? To this body? To this doorway that leads further inside of you?

See if you can now reach further inside of yourself for a moment with your eyes closed. Imagine yourself descending downward into your own body. Can you open your ear to the great below? You don't need to hear or know anything in particular yet. Trust that your calling will guide you. Trust that this wise, mysterious part of you deep within holds all the answers you need.

Notice what you feel and what thoughts or images come to you. Take your time here with some slow, deep breaths. Enjoy the treasures of the dark. The Goddess always takes her time.

When you feel ready, slowly open your eyes and begin to write.

JOURNAL PROMPTS

What about Inanna's story of descent speaks to your life? In what ways do you feel the call to descend deeper into yourself? What is calling you deep from within? What is the cost of ignoring this calling and continuing to live life as you know it? In what ways are you relying on the external world and approval from others to fill the hole inside of you? Who and what do you give your power and voice over to? Imagine passing through seven gates like Inanna, giving away something you don't need at each one; these are things that might impede your "coming home" process (self-doubt, a relationship, a job, substance use, and so on). What are those things for you? In other words, what in you needs to "die"?

EXERCISE 2:

Inanna takes her journey to the underworld to reclaim all the parts of her that have not been "allowed." She is told that women who travel below will not return, but she goes anyway, guided by the voice inside.

Inanna senses that she has wounds that need to be tended, and she experiences feelings that have not been felt before. She intuits the need to embody her dark sister Ereshkigal, rather than flee from difficult emotions and circumstances. She must let the entirety of the human experience swarm within her. As she begins to reclaim all parts of herself, she also reclaims her power, her voice, and her wholeness. She no longer fears herself. She is unapologetically clear about who she truly is.

JOURNAL PROMPTS

Take some time to think about your shadow parts, those which you've hidden away for one reason or another. When working with these more challenging areas of ourselves, it is always important to bring forth cherishing Mother love, which is manifested by unconditional acceptance and compassion for all that you are and ever have been. The cherishing Mother adores you, no matter what. You can do no "right" or "wrong" in her eyes. Allow the energy of unconditional love to hold you as you reflect on the following:

What is "unlovable" about you?

What parts of you feel rejected?

Where do you feel cast out or exiled?

What parts of you feel scary?

Where or how do you feel ugly?

What parts are not allowed to show in your "real life"?

Where do you feel "not enough"? These are the dark feminine parts of yourself that have been exiled. Try to observe with compassion and curiosity as you learn about and reclaim your wholeness. Here are a few more questions to consider: What unexpressed desires do you have?

What unlived dream do you harbor?

What unexpressed lust do you feel?

What unexpressed rage do you hold?

What unprocessed grief do you carry?

What ugliness do you long to express?

What power have you buried or repressed?

How can you safely begin to honor and express all these parts of yourself? What would you need to feel comfortable doing this?

UnMothered

It's one thing to have had a mother. It's an-
other thing to have been Mothered.
If you were only tolerated and never celebrated
Your work is to celebrate yourself.
Your job is joy.
Run from toleration.
Run toward celebration.
You are worth celebrating.
Let that sink into your cells.

The most important lens through which to see the
wounded Maiden is always going to be compassion.
Typically, when women are in the stage of wounded Maiden, they
respond to a painful experience, like abandonment, rejection,
neglect, shame, or scarcity. To address her needs, she needs
to be approached with love and compassionate inquiry, yet
so often, she receives scolding and berating, which make her
wounds worse.

We find core wounds at the center of the Maiden stories. Finding them is vital if we are to become Mother because, when we tell the story, we become the narrator, and we have agency to change. No longer are we the subject or victim.

As the creator of the story, we change our perspective so we can observe and grow, instead of agonizing and stagnating. We see a character who has wounds and flaws. When we tell these wounded Maiden stories with compassion for ourselves, we move beyond her wounds and set the stage for a new story.

The only way to write a new story in your life is to expel everything about the old story so the old plot lines don't drive the new ones. Storytelling is the teaching method of any sacred rite of passage, where we teach from the body—and not from books. We teach from the wisdom that has been growing in our bones. Telling my story, identifying my wounds, and then responding to them with compassion have been key elements of my own path to Mother.

I haven't had my biological mother in my life for twenty-four years. She was named Elizabeth, and she was a diminutive, pretty woman with soft, thin blonde hair, and she died from lung cancer three weeks after I turned seventeen. She was forty-five and had been sick for four years.

Before that, we never got along well: we just couldn't agree on much. We lived in the same house, but we were a million miles apart. I believed I was just a mirror into which she did not want to look.

One time, my mother curled up in bed next to me—a rare instance of her seeking connection. I wanted to touch her, lying there so close, but I felt frozen and afraid. The energy between us was all disconnected awkwardness, failed interactions, and shattered expectations. She only stayed a short moment. I was frozen in that bed, wanting to say all the things caught in my heart, but I couldn't. Instead, I found myself caught in the clutches of the unfinished story of her life.

Nearly half my clients say they longed for a "present" mother. That when she was actually physically there, she was a million miles away. That longing for a disconnected mother is what brings many of us here, now. We didn't experience the unconditional love and acceptance of the woman who birthed us, because she had unhealed Maiden wounds that never allowed her to become Mother. This is the core wound of being unMothered.

She had been stifled in her career and passed that wound along to me. She became pregnant with my twin sister and me at age twenty-five, just after landing a job at *Glamour* magazine. Before that, she had worked at the now-defunct *Mademoiselle*. When she became a mother unexpectedly, she felt she needed to quit her job for a simple life, and my family moved to Charlottesville, Virginia.

I always hated that she felt she had to do that for us. I imagined her resentment toward me and even resented myself for being the cause of her aborted dream. When I never received the attention, love, or understanding from her I so desired, I made it my mission to impress her to get that attention and make her proud. I was trying to heal her wound by earning her approval. This was my wound of unworthiness. I felt that I had to redeem my mother's unlived ambition to prove my worth to her.

I remember once telling her, "When I grow up, I'm going to work at a magazine in New York City too."

My mother said, "Oh, there are only a few magazines in New York City. Why don't you shoot a little lower?" My spirit fell to the ground, deflated. I never really knew why she said that, but I never forgot it either.

I felt dismissed and ashamed, and vowed to work at *Rolling Stone* as my first job. I had been obsessed with magazines for years. I lined issues of *Sassy, Jane, Spin,* and *Rolling Stone* on my bedroom shelves meant for books. I carefully reviewed all the copies that had piled up on my bureau and bedside table and crept down the hall into the family room.

Rolling Stone married my two passions: music, which I loved so much I pasted up every inch of my bedroom walls with song lyrics, and journalism, which I viewed as a chance to peer into a famous person's private world and open them up intimately for one rare moment. *Rolling Stone* was my grail at the time, and I chose to run toward it like my hair was on fire.

My sister had a different experience—she had always been closer to my mother and didn't feel the pain of alienation in adolescence. But we both suffered when my father left that same year when our parents decided to divorce.

With my father gone, I turned my back on my mother, even though she had just been diagnosed with lung cancer and began spending most of her time in bed. I've worked with lots of women who do the same. They reject the feminine as a defense mechanism. They witness weakness, emotionality, addiction, or smallness, and their survival instincts choose the father even if the father doesn't choose them.

For the four years she was sick, I carried on as if nothing was happening. That fantasy stole my precious final time with my mother. In the face of the power of her inevitable death, I played pretend. And when it was time for the end, I was not at all prepared. There were no do-overs, even if I have wished for them every day since. This was my core wound of regret.

Once, during her last days, I came home from school to find her suffering alone in bed. She felt terrible, had lost all her hair, and had shrunk to half her original size. I mustered my courage, terrified of saying the wrong thing, looking for the right words. I said, "I love you, Mom. I'm sorry you're sick."

She looked at me, skeptical, doubtful, and said, "Do you really mean that?" And I shook.

"Yes," I said, my voice quivering. But now I wasn't sure either. Because of the deep insecurity as a result of my unMothered-ness, I always shivered when my truth was in question. After that moment, when my mother questioned my goodness and my truth, I never believed in myself or trusted what I felt. This lack of self-love became another wound.

My mother died in the hospital on January 10, 1997, at five o'clock in the afternoon. On our way home to our motherless house, the sky moaned, and lightning cracked through the snow, electrifying the clouds. We stopped to look up at the show, our heads tossed back and our icy breath visible in the air. For a moment, we were afraid of nothing. The worst had happened, and blood still ran through our veins, breath still filled our lungs, and that was all that we knew. I remember it looked like the lights were flickering in heaven.

I went into my mother's room at home, and I fell into her closet, where I used to hide from the world in the dark. I put on her clothes, a pair of black silk pants and a tight blue-and-black striped cotton sweater, that still smelled like her perfume. I then went upstairs, and I laid on my bed. I remember I had no underwear on because no one had done laundry in our house for weeks, or maybe months. I laid in my bed, and I cried, "Mom, if you come back, I promise to hate myself." I had no concept of compassion or acceptance.

As I cried out, "Mom, Mom, Mom," suddenly there were two hands, one beneath my back, and one under the backs of my knees. I was held in a sweet embrace and relieved to be, just so briefly, not alone. Without my mother for the first time in my life, I felt the love of the Great Mother, the divine feminine, but I didn't know what it was. Because the Mother was buried so deeply in our culture, I had no idea who or what was in the room with me. Only that I needed it, desperately.

My desire to receive my mother's approval and praise continued to fuel me. On spring break from my senior year in college in Virginia, when all the other kids seemed to be interviewing at reputable jobs in finance or business, I loitered in the lobby of *Rolling Stone* until the managing editor, Bob Love, left his office. I recognized him from the videos I'd stayed up late to watch in the university library instead of studying for exams. I followed him into the elevator, gave a nervous but infinitely rehearsed pitch on why I was meant to work at *Rolling Stone*. He took me to coffee, where I told him of my passion and knowledge of the magazine, as well as the story about my mother, and he gave me a summer internship.

The office environment turned out to be the ultimate boy's club. I would walk past the editors' closed glass doors where they'd gather a few times a day, feeling totally left out and insecure. They were so confident and exclusive; their space was a locker room of conspiratorial whispers and loud laughter, with cigarettes and tumblers of whiskey. I would understand later that most interns are on the outside of the action, but at that point, I took it personally.

Five years later, when I met the man who would become my fiancé, Tim, in that East Village bar, my mother's burning journalism dream was down to a cold ember. This was terrifying and confusing—and snuffed my ambition. So I did what I would do back then when I felt fear: run and numb. I had bounced around to five rock journalism jobs in four years, and my drinking, which started with my mother's death, was growing worse. I knew this was unhealthy. I knew I had no guidance.

In wounded Maiden, we live life like fugitives, starting fires and fleeing them, burning bridges in every direction we run. We try on masks and fantasy roles. If you think about the Maiden archetypally as a beginning phase, this makes sense. She lives for the fresh and the new, guided by her young, foolish heart to leap off unknown cliffs. And this is necessary because we must learn from our adventurous experiences. But the Maiden can only begin things. She has yet to cultivate the nurturing consistency of the archetypal Mother, to see things through to completion.

She aborts the process every time. She bites off more than she can chew and makes promises she can't honor. She's always looking for herself through external validation, not inner value. She abandons others before they can abandon her.

Not having responded to her soul calling yet, there's no path to follow, and she often ends up getting lost in the woods. And because she's young, the Maiden believes time is endless, and so she wastes it. What is needed is compassion and recognition that Maiden time is about her search to become her full self. She must become someone who roots and rises to offer her authentic contributions. Yet if she hasn't developed her confidence and has instead accumulated a collection of Maiden wounds, she will continually seek approval and acceptance. She cannot give herself these. She will remain in the bud and unbloomed, a girl in a woman's body. She will also play the victim, dwelling in self-pity while seeking sympathy from others for her misfortunes. She mistakes this sympathy for love and never rises out of her victimhood.

Compassion is the key to disrupting this pattern. Until we radically accept ourselves, we won't make it out of this endless loop.

Until we approve of ourselves, we are always going to feel and act like we have to prove our worth and lovability. This compassion must also extend out to other wounded Maidens that we know. They are everywhere because our culture celebrates the Maiden for her beauty and youth and ignores the power and wisdom of the Mother. The culture sexualizes and desires the Maiden and de-sexualizes and rejects the Mother. The bias against women in middle age actually makes the Maiden afraid to age and mature and motivates her to stay stuck. Yet the ancient archetypes of the feminine offered a different vision, one that we can reorient toward now to restore our birthright as whole women.

Archetypes are universal symbols, images, and constructs that help us make sense of our individual lives. The psychoanalyst Carl Jung introduced the term in an essay he wrote in 1919 called "Instinct and the Unconscious."[6] Before he termed them "archetypes," he referred to "primordial images." These are collective characters and patterns in the myths of our lives that become the keys to make sense of our lives as well. The following are the fundamental archetypes that we work with in the sacred feminine. They come to us through the ages, back from when the sacred feminine was a central aspect of human life, and are still noted and celebrated in a growing number of Goddess-loving covens and female spiritual circles emerging today.

The Child: She is the new moon, the dawn, and the midwinter Celtic celebration of Imbolc, when the ice starts to thaw and spring seeds begin pulsing to life under the earth.

The Maiden: She represents the beginning of life, morning, spring: the waxing moon, the equinox fertility festival, and the flower beginning to swell in the bud.

The Mother: She symbolizes the middle of life, the afternoon, the summer solstice, the full moon, and the flower in glorious bloom.

The Crone: She reminds us of the ending of life, the harvest, the visitations of the dead, the evening and night, the autumn and winter of the seasons, and the wilting flower returning to earth.

I want to be clear here; there is nothing "bad" or "wrong" with the archetypal Maiden in her natural, healthy state. The Maiden always lives within us, and so does the Mother, as do the Child and the Crone. Sometimes you feel like a child, and sometimes you feel like a grown-up, and sometimes you feel like a wise old woman. That's natural because we carry all these archetypes within, like stacking Russian dolls. These energies don't die or go away—and one will always be more prominent at certain times in your life.

The Maiden in her natural and healthy presentation is awesome and vital. She is bold, courageous, daring, adventurous, and joyful. She is everything you feel and think about spring. When I summon Maiden energy in my body, I see a young woman in the morning, running barefoot through a field of flowers, her hair flying in the wind. There is a wild sense of innocence and the rush of new life.

The archetypal Maiden is fresh, eager, excited, expansive, unfolding, joyful, becoming, exploring, and ready for life's adventure. She is also not yet mature—she has yet to reach the more advanced stage of mental and emotional development that is characteristic of an adult.

The development into maturity happens over a long time. While it takes integrating the experiences of one's life, it also requires consciousness. Simply aging does not bring maturity. Author, storyteller, and activist for the dying Stephen Jenkinson is a champion of maturity and elderhood for our culture. He teaches and writes about how to return "the skills of deep living to our culture."[7] He says that to mature, we must engage with aging; it is not a passive process. It is the Mother's work to engage with her process of growing older, while the Maiden is still in the collecting and experiencing stage.

What goes wrong is that women present themselves primarily as Maiden when we're meant to be in Mother. But this is not our fault. This is the fault of a culture that has lost its soul and connection to the sacred feminine archetypes. The life source of humanity's culture went underground with the Goddess when she was suppressed. With the death of ritual, which was once woven into the fabric of life, came the death of our wholeness and maturity.

As I look at these white roses above my computer, shining in full bloom, I think about how these flowers came to be. I think about their roots, deep into the soil. It is that connection to the earth—to the earth of their bodies and the body of the earth—that made it possible for them to trust the process of pushing up through the dark confinements of their buds and opening to their glory.

The world needs its strong, receptive, open-to-life Mothers. Let's gather ourselves and answer our own cries, for only then can we answer the cries of a burning world.

Reflection Exercise: Maiden Reactions and Mother Responses

In Maiden, life happens to us. In Mother, life happens through us. In many ways, the wounded Maiden traits appear as opposites to the traits of the Mother. The Maiden reacts, while the Mother responds with creativity. In a few chapters, I will walk you through a meditation to meet your Maiden. Still, before we do that, it is helpful to further understand the characteristics found in wounded Maiden and the opposites of those characteristics, which are how the Mother archetype responds. Below is a chart of examples of wounded Maiden traits with their corresponding Mother responses. I've listed several here for you, with a few spaces left at the bottom for you to play with by filling in some of your Maiden reactions and their Mother responses. This exercise aims to begin to develop the awareness of your reactions and the understanding that you can transform them into responses.

MAIDEN REACTIONS	MOTHER RESPONSES
"I am sick of feeling..."	"I am ready to feel..." or "I want to feel..."
Insecure	Inner security
Reactionary	Responsive
Not present, always busy	Present, living for the moment
Victimization and self-pity	Responsible for my life
The need to seek approval from others	Inner wholeness and love
The need to please others	Self-love and acceptance
Terror and panic	Safety and security
Inauthentic	Unapologetically myself
The urge to consume	Creative
That what happens is about me	What happens is always about love
I must wait to be saved	I can save myself
I bite off more than I can chew	I take what I can handle and what I want

Depressed	Joyful
I suck all the air out of the room	I hold the room with confidence
Fear	Trust
Jealous of and competitive with other women	Supportive of other women
Seeks answers outside myself	Self-sourced
Others can't help	Worthy of receiving help
Self-care is selfish	Self-care is sacred
Desperate for attention	Content and at ease
I need to ask others for permission	I ask the Goddess within
Perfectionism	Fluidity and nonlinear growth
Agitation and irritation	Peace
Full room and empty, lonely soul	Empty room and full soul

I must give to get	I give to heal the world
Addiction and self-sabotage	Sobriety and self-advocacy
Overwhelmed	In charge
Not-enough-ness	I have enough, I am enough

JOURNAL PROMPTS

What else would you add to the list of what you're "sick of feeling"? And what would be the "Mother response" to your list?

What are your core Maiden wounds?

Can you identify how and when you developed these wounds?

What Maiden reactions do you have that come from these wounds?

How could you respond more like Mother when your Maiden wounds are triggered?

Is there someone in your life who regularly demonstrates Mother responses? Can you find ways to spend more time with this person?

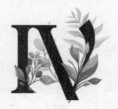

Time in the Underworld

Who am I to be blue?
Look at my family and fortune, look
at my friends and my house.
Who am I to feel deadened?
Who am I to feel spent?
Look at my health and my money.
Where do I go to feel good? Why
do I still look outside me?
Clearly, I've seen it won't work.

ALANIS MORISSETTE[8]

By the time my fiancé Tim decided to leave me, I was in the grip of an addiction I couldn't escape and a depression I couldn't shake. I had become the substance-abuse cliché, popping Valium pills between glasses of wine, overflowing in my once-glamorous dresses because I never exercised anymore. Tim had become numb to my constant vacillation between indulgence and remorse. One time we were out drinking with a friend in the East Village, and she became alarmed when I had one of my panic attacks between drink rounds. I remember that Tim just rolled his eyes. "She always does this," he murmured to her, "these cries for help."

I didn't know that it was possible to stop partying. I didn't know how to take care of myself. I didn't know how to mother myself. I didn't know then that you can hold and heal yourself.

Sometimes my Mother spirit now rises to find my lost Maiden, still somewhere out in the night, and hovers over her, wraps her arms around her, picks her up off the dirty street corner, takes her home, and tucks her in and tells her everything's gonna be all right.

But back then, at thirty years old, I was a hot mess. Dumped from my relationship and sacked from my job. *Loser* is a hard word. But it made sense: yes, I had lost it all. I still had my dog, Gracie, who was like a shepherd for a lost sheep. Yet she did allow me one moment of heroics that helped jolt me out of my life stupor.

We were walking down a wooded road, and Gracie was trotting by my side without a leash. Out of nowhere, a woman with two leashed, growling, frantic dogs appeared in front of us. I heard Gracie growl—she was a rescue dog who didn't back down from a fight.

The woman screamed: "They're not friendly!"

Gracie started to rush past me. With my eyes on the dogs ahead, in one swift stroke, my hand shot down and grabbed my dog by the neck scruff, stopping her in midair. With fast-moving Mother instinct, I responded, and everyone was safe. For one moment, in a time when I usually caused the storm, I was the shelter.

For years I would remember that moment.

That's who I really was underneath the disarray I'd created with my addictions and fantasies. I was a natural Mother, a wild woman with brave, ferocious instincts, a queen of her realm. But I had been waiting for permission and initiation to be strong.

The most frightened we ever feel is when we feel totally alone. Isolation makes us sick and connection heals us. *Am I the only one who thinks and feels this? Then I must be crazy!* and that's horrifying.

But how do we connect with that source?

My reaction was always to retreat to the oblivion that drugs and alcohol offered so I could avoid that question. After one chaotic drug-and-alcohol-infused night with a man whose name I had already forgotten, I woke up more remorseful and ashamed than I had ever felt. On my knees, through heaving tears, I blurted out, "Is anyone there? I cannot take one more step on this path. If there is anyone there, please help me to live or help me to die."

Shortly thereafter, a soft white light filled the room. It looked like a cloudy puff of cotton candy. Although shaken, I stumbled to my feet and wobbled like a newborn foal to look in the mirror. I was shocked at what I saw. My hair looked soft despite years of bleach and extensions abuse, and it fell in angelic, bouncy waves. My eyes had gone from murky blue to piercing violet; my pupils looked like hearts.

I could see white energy flowing from my hands, and when I walked out to the open field behind my rented cabin, I was greeted by the vision of a massive woman in white, floating above the grass. She said she was the Goddess.

"I have saved you," she told me. "And now you serve me." I understood her to mean that I would now turn my focus from seeking escape toward serving the greater purposes of creativity, joy, unconditional love, the Earth, and the source of all being.

She embodied the healing, magical, feminine energy I felt I had been missing since I felt the Great Mother's embrace on my mother's bed after she died. My introduction to this power was abrupt and disorienting—as I would hear from many women with similar experiences, when the Goddess rearranges your life, she disorients you to reorient you.

I can see how you would surmise it was induced by the night before's Klonopin and wine. Yet, I choose to see this as a moment of pure grace that defies rationality. And that Kundalini awakening would alter the course of my life and the intensity of the awakening would continue for months.

Now, I see my time abusing substances as part of my journey to the underworld. I hadn't yet learned that the underworld is also the place of rebirth. I longed for an escape, to return home to the Mother, to the garden where I was from and where I once belonged.

The underworld is also place of mourning: it's where one's no-longer-useful life goes to die before the new one can be born. It's where you go to honor and grieve the life of the Maiden. It's the limbo space between the Maiden and the Mother.

In Inanna's story, when she descends through the gates of the underworld, the gatekeepers tell her, "The rules of the underworld are perfect." At each gate, they strip her of another worldly possession. Women on this journey through the Maiden to Mother experience big aha moments when they hear this because initiation into the underworld is always marked by loss. And that loss can appear in a myriad of ways, such as:

Loss of a job.

Loss of a dream.

Loss of a relationship.

Loss of a home.

Loss of a loved one.

Loss of health.

Loss of identity.

We find our way into the underworld by getting lost, by accident. We experience a painful absence of something we deem vital, and we go down there to find it. The light in our life has gone out, and we are plunged into the darkness.

But no matter how the invitation from the underworld is worded, no matter the paper stock or calligraphy, it will invite you to a crossroads. You will be stuck with a heavy, life-changing choice.

But the only way we get out of the dark is first to recognize that we are in it. Although it appears frightening, this is precisely where we are meant to be. By the time we reach the belly of the Earth, the upperworld—the physical and material life we have grown accustomed to and perhaps too comfortable in—has ripped open in a great earthquake. We have fallen through the cracks, down to the belly below.

When we are in the underworld living as the wounded Maiden, we feel fragile and incapable because we don't have a framework for what is happening. Time stops for us to face ourselves. Yet, entering the terrifyingly dark underworld can be one of the most transformational gifts of your life.

When we are on our knees, paused in a dark moon phase of our life, we become undone. Like Inanna, we are being stripped of the robes we've been wearing, and we are being exposed down to the soul. To pass through the underworld, we must address the wounds of our Maiden life. We will also have to mourn the death of our Maiden.

Down here on our knees, we are calling to Goddess. Or is it she who is calling us? They are one and the same: the Goddess within us is calling on us to express her, out in the world. The beauty of falling to your knees and crying out for her help is that she answers. The work is to walk with her not just in dark times, but to walk hand in hand with her back up to the light.

Despite the terrifying events, which may have led to finding ourselves in the underworld, it is a gift to retreat and reset down there. To walk one more step on a path that wasn't ours would have been a waste of our gifts, and a waste of our lives. The underworld is where we remember who we are and what we came here to do. When we do rise, we rise with remembrance and purpose.

After that day that the Goddess visited me, I am thankful that I weaned myself off the myriad pills I was taking and never took them again. But I needed something else to fall back on in my difficult times; I had yet to develop a regimen of self-care.

One day at the local general store where I was living at the time, someone mentioned they were about to do a yoga training at the Kripalu Center in the Berkshires of Massachusetts. When I looked up the website, I saw that the center offered a lot of trainings in transformational and spiritual practices.

I had some money saved up from when my mother died, which I decided to use as a spiritual trust. I enrolled in energy healing and yoga courses at Kripalu for a few months. While I had slept through my university courses, I had a voracious appetite for this spiritual knowledge. I'd spend hours in the bookstore poring over texts and would often practice what I was learning in the center's spacious halls and gardens. They called the center "The Mothership" because it was a hub for spiritual seekers, and I felt like I belonged.

It was here that I first began learning about Inanna and understood the importance of her journey for our times. What makes Inanna so powerful for women raised on fairy tales is that her story shows a woman saving herself. In most mythology, men play the savior role.

Maureen Murdock, the author of *The Heroine's Journey*, puts a different spin on Joseph Campbell's account of the (male) hero mythology, *The Hero with a Thousand Faces*, which has since become a template for the psychological and spiritual development of the individual. Campbell's hero struggles against his father, fights adversaries, endures trials and fires, receives supernatural guidance, and eventually attains the object of his quest and settles down with a wife. It's no surprise that this journey has little to do with the female experience. The heroine's quest involves wrestling with a primal mother and overcoming ingrained social roles of subservience. In Murdock's book, she describes how the heroine begins her quest by trying to achieve success in patriarchal institutions, which leads to her deep self-questioning when she doesn't feel fulfilled. She wants something more out of life.[9] Then she experiences a spiritual death, finally recovering the power of the sacred feminine through an inner soul quest.

This all rang true for me, and when I read the myth of Inanna, I realized I wasn't alone in my desire for something more, despite having what the dominant culture told me should be enough. Now I know, after years of Maiden-to-Mother work, that this myth speaks universally to women walking the bridge into the mature feminine. They're being guided and called by the overriding sense that they're not whole. That something is desperately missing in their lives. The eco-feminist witch Starhawk wrote, "The test of a true myth is that each time you return to it, new insights and interpretations arise."[10] Every time a woman reads the myth of Inanna, she finds the gift of a new insight into her own life.

But the "more" a woman seeks at this crossroads isn't material accumulation. In fact, she may need to shed most of her belongings. She wants more of her own truth, along with more love, depth, aliveness, and adventure. Yet when she first hears her individual, inner dream, no one else will understand it. It will be up to her alone to follow it and to birth it. Your primary task is to believe in this dream, and your secondary task is to not ask other people to believe in it for you.

They will never make it come true, because you're the only one who can.

After I read the myth of Inanna, I felt I was being guided into an underworld journey. Culturally, the Goddess was still very much buried, and I would need to unearth her.

I wrote down the traits that had made me feel so disempowered, and as it happened, they were the same traits I saw in other women that made me recoil. The list went something like this:

TRAITS I AM READY TO RELEASE:

Jealousy • Insecurity • Reactivity • Fear
Scarcity • Vanity • Inauthenticity

Sycophancy • Neediness • Self-Loathing
Selfishness • Fragility • Smallness

On the other side of the paper, I wrote down the traits I wanted to replace these with.

TRAITS I AM READY TO EMBODY

Confidence • Security • Responsiveness
Safety • Enough-ness

Self-approval • Authenticity • Integrity
Wholeness • Self-loving

Generosity • Self-sourced

The trait ritual felt like an initiation; it was a beginning. It was my way of saying to Spirit, the Universe, or Goddess, "I am ready."

"Goddess Inanna," I begged, "please make a woman out of me. I am ready to release these immature traits. They are killing me. Please take them from me. Please replace them with these traits of maturity. I am ready to walk them. I am ready to be a woman."

I lit candles on the bedside tables. I imagined these were my Maiden's funeral rites, and I laid back down in my big white bed and self-attended the funeral rites of my unhealthy Maiden.

I imagined I was holding flowers, singing hauntingly as I lay down to drown in a river, surrounded by the quiet woods. I was deadly serious about change, about transformation.

That night of ritual proved to be just the beginning of the Maiden-to-Mother passage. The word *spiritual* combines the words *spirit* and *ritual*. I needed to involve my spirit in a ritual to honor this moment, to signal I was 100 percent present and ready for this transformation.

I've been studying and working with this spirit journey ever since. I've learned that when you acknowledge your greatest wound, it can become your greatest gift to others. But first it causes pain. To become a teacher or a healer, you must first survive your initiation.

Yet what our inner voice might tell us during this process has the potential to shatter life as we know it. When we're the wounded Maiden, other voices are louder than our inner voice. It can be hard to hear ourselves over the chaos of the outside drama. When we're in Mother, the inner voice is louder than the outside voice and clears the path to peace and purpose. A woman takes the heroine's journey to heal herself and offer her healed self to the world.

I need to be clear that my spiritual crisis was also a mental health crisis. I have struggled with depression and anxiety since I was a teen. While I chose to follow a spiritual path for my healing, I have also consulted therapists and doctors in my quest to become whole and have engaged in various treatments at different times in my life.

I see spirituality and mental health as intertwined because they both stem from our disconnection from ourselves, each other, and the planet. To be severed from the Earth and nature's cycles and isolated from deep self-connection naturally leads to deeper and more complex mental health issues for many. What might be medically diagnosed as depression, anxiety, bipolar, or dissociative personality disorder is also a profound recognition of this state of disconnection. In short, women can feel "crazy" living in a patriarchy. We aren't rewarded financially for our gifts of caring, the institutions of society do not equally address our emotions and health issues, and we are subjected to unrealistic expectations set by men about how we should look and act. These injustices and others put us into a permanent state of "less than" in relation to men. If we don't heal our spiritual wounds, and address how we have suffered under patriarchy, it's reasonable to expect that any mental health issues we may have will continue to plague us.

Every psychological illness can be understood as an initiation, which you must find your way through.

To become Mother, we must move from a life based on how things look to how things feel. That has been difficult until now because we have yet to truly know ourselves in wounded Maiden, so how do we know how we truly feel? Not yet knowing is exactly what the seeking phase, the *becoming* time, of the Maiden is for. The full moon needed the waxing moon to become whole; the blooming flower needed the bud; the summer was preceded by spring. And you need the Maiden to become the Mother.

You've been in search of your purpose, your identity, your place in the world. Seeking these out can become the most important work of your life. We must hear ourselves, take our own Mother advice, and spring back to life. Our true voice, the voice of our internal Mother, will guide us there.

I'm still hung up
On that last man in my bed
The one who left me
For dead
Hung up
Like Inanna on the meat hook in the underworld
Draining her blood
To die and rise whole
To lose everything but
Her soul
Only the fearless know what I mean
When you finally die to the princess
And rise the Queen.

Reflection Exercise: An Overview of the Underworld

I often say: "When I witness a woman 'really let herself go,' I trust she's descending into the underworld, to the belly of the buried, dark, and powerful feminine within. I know that what looks like insanity can mean that she's touching true sanity for the first time."

While every woman's underworld experience will be unique, count on similarities. Here are some things you can most likely expect from time in the underworld.

- We become more comfortable with the thresholds of our life stages. We are "in between" worlds, as we are no longer a Maiden and not yet a Mother.

- We become more comfortable with the death-rebirth cycle as it becomes clear that old life must die to make way for the new.

- At points we may feel "lost" in the underworld. We appreciate that getting lost is how we become found.

- We dare to see in the dark. We learn to be guided by the subtle lights, as well as our inner senses, such as our intuition and psychic knowing.

- Our inner voice grows, and the voices of the outer world fade.

- We become skilled at sorting out what parts of ourselves need to die and what parts need to be enlivened.

- We learn that we must cherish all the parts of ourselves, all our emotions, all that we yearn for, all that we have lived and learned.

- The artful skill of transforming wounds, pain, and joys into gifts and wisdom is learned and valued.

- Our outer lives may not change, or they may change dramatically. Nonetheless, we know deep inner healing is occurring.

- We begin to gain further insights about what we came here to do in this life.

EXERCISE 1:
Transforming Wounds
into Joy

Part of the medicine of the underworld is to learn to transform wounds into gifts, as well as capture all our joys and successes. Take a few minutes to reflect on the forks and turns you've taken in your life and how each one offered you a sacred gift of deeper knowing. Here are a few prompts to get you started:

1. What have been your greatest regrets, heartbreaks, failures, or losses in your life, and what have you learned from them?

2. Recall one that you listed above and imagine a gift being handed to you from this experience and placed inside of you. What would be a few words to describe that gift?

3. Now reflect on all your joys in your life. What have been your best adventures? Friendships? Successes in life or career?

4. What do you love most about yourself and your life? What are the strengths and qualities you appreciate in yourself?

5. Take a look at what you've answered for questions 3 and 4 and imagine these are beautiful gifts that have been handed to you. What have you learned from them?

EXERCISE 2:
Letting Go of What Needs Letting Go with a Water Renewal Ceremony

Slow down and come into your body. Take three deep breaths and close your eyes. Imagine you are sitting at the bank of a beautiful, clear river that flows down into a valley of lush greens and blues. As you sit quietly, take in the sound of the water rushing along the rocks, as the sky's clouds roll overhead.

As you center yourself, identify one thing you know you need to let go of, something that needs to "die-off"—that no longer serves you. Imagine this thing coming from your belly. Feel the aching to let it go and for it no longer to be a part of you. Once you know what is ready to be released, imagine placing it into your hands as you sit near the river. When you are ready, say your goodbyes and gently place it into the river as you watch it wash away and out of your sight. Know that the river can hold it for you from this day forward as you say, whisper, or sing the following words:

"I thank you for the lessons that have
brought me here to this day.
I now release you and let you wash away
May the pain leave,
And may only the wisdom stay."

When you feel ready to repeat, do so again as many times as you need to offer up what needs to go. You may need to repeat this exercise dozens (maybe hundreds) of times working on the same topic again and again until it really, once and for all, washes away.

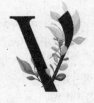

Excavating the Exiled You

Remember the fairy tales that keep you
from reuniting with the sacred feminine?
They told you, "Don't go into the dark woods.
You'll find a witch, and she will kill you."
But they were trying to throw you
off the path of your power.
You must go into the dark woods.
You must find the witch.
She will be you and she will save you.

Here's what I've told you about Inanna, the Queen of Heaven and Earth: She hears Ereshkigal, her dark sister, separated from Inanna in the underworld, crying out in grief at the death of her husband. In that instant, Inanna knows what she has to do.

Calls from the soul are like having an internal phone that rings in a tone only you can hear. It's not going to stop ringing, no matter how hard you try to ignore it. When Inanna's soul phone rang, she answered. Inanna said: "I'm going to the underworld because this is my calling."

Every wounded Maiden has a buried self, or an Ereshkigal, who is trying to connect with her. We've severed the dark parts, or the wild pieces, of ourselves in order to survive in a conformist culture. As early as most of us can recall, our wild child was forced to wear a nice-girl sheep suit over her wolf body. She was never allowed to tell the sometimes uncomfortable truths of how she really felt. Eventually, she became—and her life became—a lie. She walks in disguise. And the disguise works—certainly for others, who felt comfortable around her pleasantries and niceties—until at last, the costume began to suffocate her.

Who is your Ereshkigal?

She's all the parts of you that you haven't let anyone see. And these are killing you. Chances are, since you were young, you've hidden the stranger, wilder you and offered the world instead the safe version of you: this is the false self. The work we do in the underworld is to become reacquainted with the abandoned, hidden parts of us that have withered in our personal basements until now. These parts are "dark" because they haven't been brought into the light and because they haven't been felt and expressed. Every time these aspects have begun to emerge, you've shoved them back down, terrified that to express them could mean being exiled, rejected, or abandoned. The irony is that as you've modified your behavior in fear of rejection, you've only rejected yourself. And when rejected, these feelings will fester and grow. They'll grow until their fierce growl shocks you into awareness. If you continue to ignore them, they'll stop begging for your attention, and they begin to eat at you from the inside. The true you never bloomed, she was crushed before she could do so. She is Ereshkigal, exiled to your underworld. She is the exiled you.

When you gather up the parts of you that you haven't felt safe to embody or express—your rage, grief, and fear, and the full range of your sexuality—you will become whole again. These are your powers, not your liabilities. You can protect yourself from wounding your Maiden further by letting these feelings out when you feel them. We imagine that protection comes from an outside source, but the truth is that we are the guardians of our own safety. Once we reclaim ourselves, we understand that others' responses and reactions to us are theirs to hold. The fear of rejection doesn't motivate us as it once did, and we feel freer to let the most powerful emotions work their way through us, up to the dimension of expression. Our work in the process of blooming is to see, to hear, to honor, to love, to embody, and to express all of ourselves.

You'd think that the cry of your inner Ereshkigal would have been impossible to ignore. To ignore one's intuition is not just to abandon one's own voice and power, but also to abandon the voice of the Earth and the Great Mother Goddess. When a woman abandons her true self, she loses her ability to hear her truth, she loses access to her self-guidance and protection, and she loses access to her vitality and a real life. The community loses her healing. If she has children, they lose a powerful mother to guard them; if she has a partner, they lose the erotic and sensual; her friends lose an ally; and the Earth loses its advocacy.

Instead, we have become gold-medal Olympians in the art of self-betrayal. We are brilliant at ignoring our voices and needs in place of someone else's. We numb ourselves in addiction. We feel something uncomfortable, and instead of actively listening to it and leaning into its plea for attention, we stuff it down. And all the while, we are dying, and the Earth is dying from our disconnected relationship to ourselves and to the Earth. Without the tools of self-witnessing, self-love, and self-mothering, we perpetuate this deadly disconnect.

I know now that I was a product of the fairy tales that were programmed into so many of us as young girls. *Rapunzel, Cinderella, Sleeping Beauty, Snow White*. All the Maidens waited helplessly.

This is early "princessization," the conditioning of girls to stay meek and to fear their own power. Princessization keeps us out of trouble, especially the good kind of trouble that can change the world. It conditions us to be passive, pretty, and pleasing.

Of course, at the time of this writing, there are better modern princesses for children today. There are *Frozen*'s Anna and Elsa—Elsa is sovereign and powerful, and Anna is adventurous and funny. There is Moana, a brave Polynesian princess-warrior who answers the call to adventure into a different life from the one she was born into. There is courageous and independent Merida from *Brave*, who actually contends for, and wins, her own hand in marriage. Yet most of you reading this did not have those strong examples as young girls. I myself remember learning from Ariel in *The Little Mermaid* that if you're really pretty and quiet, the prince will choose you over the bad witch, and your father will pass you off at sixteen from his hands to your husband's.

At thirty-three years old, I was still princessized; trapped like Snow White, suffocating inside of a glass coffin. The coffin was lined with mirrors and selfies and others' perceptions and opinions of me, and I continued to add to the collage. I was the center of my own universe, a very lonely place to be. All my energy went into the external. I may have looked good, but I felt horrible.

Ereshkigal is the symbol of the wounded Maiden within us. She is the repressed and severed one who deserves our tending, our active listening, our healing, and our care. Only then might we care truly for others and the world. Only then might we have the space and capacity; only then might we serve from a healed, and not wounded, place.

The soul-knowing that we were born with is still there. Reviving it requires trusting the Mother's voice. The louder she speaks, the farther you can travel down the path that is destined just for you. Only you know who you really are and what you're really here to do. The reason you go down to the underworld is to retrieve this true you.

For some people, the underworld becomes a familiar place that stops inspiring fear. For Tamara Mihalic, who worked with me on her Maiden-to-Mother journey, the underworld offers her an opportunity to face her dark emotions head on. She told me how when she became a mother and found herself raising her son alone without her formerly abusive partner, her moods became much less resilient. "I kept telling myself that I just needed to meditate more or do more yoga and that would help me feel less mad," she said. But understanding the underworld gave her the courage to focus on and truly feel her frustration and anger. "I just became the dark Goddess in the underworld, which I now see as a quiet and dark and fertile womb where everything is born," she said. She's gotten to a place where she now embraces her time there.

Our bodies, the Goddess, and the Earth are speaking louder than ever. You could say our souls are screaming. If we are not brave enough to choose to give birth to our true life, then the repression we experience might just kill us. The call from the underworld doesn't call to end your life, but to begin it!

The soul call finds its way into our dreams. It wakes us from our sleep. It stalks us with signs and "coincidences."

Carl Jung called these meaningful coincidences "synchronicity," which he defined as "A meaningful coincidence of two or more events where something other than the probability of chance is involved . . . Synchronicity, an ever-present reality for those who have eyes to see."[11]

Synchronicity brings signs, symbols, and messages. An age-old spiritual saying is that these signs are how we know we're on our path. A woman I work with was grieving the slow illness of her mother, Iris, who was soon to die. Drawn to a new spiritual path, she was about to perform an initiation ceremony in a sacred temple. As she climbed the stairs up to the room where her supporters were gathered, another temple resident she didn't know was climbing down the stairs, carrying a giant painting of a purple iris. For this daughter, the painting was a symbol of her mother's presence, a synchronicity that blessed her initiation ceremony.

Not everyone takes to these signs so readily. Sometimes once we start to recognize synchronicities, we might want to un-see them, because they often indicate a fork in the road, and point to a new direction that we're terrified to take.

We see this looming choice in the books we're reading, in the songs we hear. We cannot escape from ourselves, from the infinite web of the Universe's connections that transmit truth to us. The harder we resist our soul call, the harder our underworld descent will be. Until we have the courage to accept this, the soul call will continue.

Interestingly enough, the story of Inanna has followed women throughout history, awakening them to their soul calling even as patriarchal oppression grew and the sacred feminine had to go into hiding. Yet the story of Inanna was passed from generation to generation, changing details and contexts, but always wrestling with the female descent into the underworld and her rebirth. She was Ishtar in Assyria, she was Salome dancing with seven veils in the Bible, and in Greco-Roman antiquity, she was the kidnapped maiden Persephone, who was forced to stay down in the underworld for half the year, triggering the winter.[12]

The passage to the underworld is one of the most powerful stories ever told, and it is eternally relevant. If we have wounded and exiled parts of ourselves, they will always be found down there in the darkest places. Reclaiming these parts that are calling out to us takes bravery and letting go of old stories. The tools laid out here in this book make this hard work of resuscitating our full selves a bit easier. Until we surrender, tired and tender, we are angry, exhausted, fragile, and tightly wound people holding onto the dying things while the new life struggles to be born within. The holding on too tightly to what we know, instead of allowing the unfolding of the unknown, is how we break. Letting go is easier said than done, but as country artist Lori McKenna sings in "You Get a Love Song," "I know the only thing harder than letting go is holding on." And like all great sages say: The holding on is tearing you apart. The letting go will carry you.

It should be noted that at this stage, we can literally become sick of ourselves. Some of us are mysteriously bedridden from unknown ailments. We're tired of pretending to be small, polite, pretty, and pleasing, and the rejection of those false identities makes us physically ill.

More than once a female friend said to me, "I don't trust you," or "I don't believe you." And in those times, they were right not to, because I had been lying to them while pretending to be their friend. I wore a pretty and pleasing mask. I was the wolf, but in sheep's clothing.

Healthy women are wolves, not sheep. When you pretend to be a sheep, you're far more dangerous than if you'd shown your fangs and outed yourself as a wolf from the get-go, than if you'd been your wild self.

The time in the underworld can transform us back into our wild selves. My experiences allowed me to reclaim my feminine power that extends through the lineage of women who have been persecuted throughout history. As I emerged, I felt more and more drawn to practices of Goddess celebration and witchcraft, long hidden in the shadows of patriarchy. In these traditions, someone who has been to the underworld, perhaps dozens of times, can help others navigate their own dark journeys and heal themselves.

Witches know that darkness is not evil; it's not the devil: it is a necessary condition that puts us in touch with our intuition, wisdom, and our ability to self-heal. To become conscious of the darkness that humans all experience means that it cannot control you anymore. To be whole, we must acknowledge, and not fear, our own shadows.

The history of witchcraft is instructional for women today who are transforming from wounded Maiden into a grounded woman who accepts her power and uses it for the good of all beings. In European lineage, long before the Vikings and the Druids, women known as wicces (pronounced "witches") engaged in oracular practices like runes; they called upon the healing powers of herbs, helped one another with fertility and childbirth, and offered transformative rituals to their communities. They were animist, believing that spirit resided inside everything, and they called upon these spirits and the Goddess life force to influence events.

When the Romans conquered Northern European territory in the seventh century CE, these practices were suppressed, and witches became vilified because powerful women had no place in a patriarchal system that prioritized domination and productivity. Women were treated like unpaid servants to men and children and could not continue to control their own reproductive lives through herbs and midwifery. Women became subordinate to men and their endeavors, which required the devaluing of their status and contributions. The witch hunts were used as a fear tactic to get women to subordinate themselves. Covens were dissolved and became illegal. (That's why witches wear black, because they had to move through the night in all black, in cloaks, and try to blend into the night.) Yet their practices never completely disappeared and have reemerged at various times over the past millennia. Even as European imperial forces spread around the globe, the colonized cultures used nature-based practices to resist domination. People banded together with underground syncretized rituals to keep their spirits vital in traditions like Cuban Santería, Brazilian Umbanda, and New Orleans Voodoo, among others.

Yet we are now seeing a resurgence of these practices in the twenty-first century.

As Amanda Yates Garcia wrote in *Initiated*, her memoir of growing up as a contemporary witch:

> The forces of patriarchal authority have destroyed our stones, our caves, our temples, our cathedrals. Turned our Goddesses into scorned women, whores. Controlled our wombs. Taken our bodies. Ignored our words. Burned us at the stake. But we are still here. Throughout history, in secret, witches have kept the fires of the divine feminine burning. Small coals, tended secretly in our caves. Our initiations are the pains of our labor. The Goddess is being reborn.[13]

Some of this is due to the work of Gerald Gardner, an early twentieth-century British amateur anthropologist and author who spent time with a secret coven and wrote about their activities and popularized a new form of the old traditions called Wicca. Gardner spent the rest of his life creating new festivals and practices that spread around the world and encouraged many individuals to develop their own relationships to the healing power of nature and the Goddess. I was one of these individuals, but at the time that I discovered the long lineage of the sacred feminine, I didn't have a coven to initiate me, or even know that there were hundreds of thousands of others embarking on a magic path.

In the spring of my feminine awakening, after I left Kripalu, I continued to open myself up to the messages from the Goddess. The words that she poured through me seemed initially crazy: they were messages of self-love and empowerment that resembled nothing anyone I knew had ever spoken of. Yet, I could tell these were also potentially helpful—maybe even healing—messages. They were very coarse at the beginning. I remember feeling like a cave woman scrawling on walls. It was no accident these words were being poured into me to be poured out to the world. The Goddess had explicitly told me I now served her purposes of love.

"How do you know when something else is speaking?" So many women would ask me in the beginning of my post-underworld effort to share my experience. I'd tell them, "It's things you can't have known, things you didn't know before they rushed into you. You've never thought these things before—it's wisdom that's expressed so much wiser and clearer—it rhymes, and it sings! The words make you feel something; they help you heal something." These words were much wiser than any words in my head before.

After ten years of communication with her, I now know how the Goddess speaks. Open any ancient book of Goddess invocations, and the words that come through rhyme and are encoded with spells—they break open to mean something else.

I became a vessel for the Goddess's wild words, streaming through my body like rivulets of electrified water.

Like so many of us, ever since I was a child, I thought witches were "bad," and ever since I was a child, I thought I was bad. I didn't know how intertwined and healing those two narratives would become.

I would come to find better and more useful answers in Goddess totems in the natural world.

I asked the spider, "Does it both-
er you they're scared of you?"
And she said, "The wise ones aren't, and the un-
wise give me a wide berth, and that works for me."
I asked the snake, and she said, "Those who
can see honor me, and that's enough for me."
I asked the wolf, and she said, "I have
great power, so they should be."

I began to understand the need for the protective aspects of the mature feminine: the spider's bite and the snake's hiss and the wolf's growl. The feminine is sacred and must be respected and protected. I know now that if we can't protect ourselves, we can't protect others.

In my childhood, my common experience was to be condemned. I was scolded, sent to my room, shamed, and exiled for anything I said that ruffled the adults' feathers. And a lot of what came from the bones and belly of me positively shook the room. Eventually, at around twelve years old, I developed a type of anxiety that channeled into a crippling fear of spiders—arachnophobia. I ended up in therapy, albeit briefly—not because I didn't need it but because there was rarely any consistency and stability in my childhood home and regularity was hard to come by.

Now I actually identify with the spider: she is the Creatrix. I recognize now that I had been afraid of myself. I realize this terror was symbolic of the severance from my dark feminine, from the parts of me that scared people and made them uncomfortable. When I see my true self, I see a woman in her power, weaving a web from the silk of my own body.

But my power, deemed dark, was disposable for everyone else. What wasn't disposable was my safety. So I buried my power and chose the safety of being tolerated over the terror of being feared. And I projected others' fears of my dark side onto the shadowy figure of the spider. That dark creative power was exactly what Inanna goes down to retrieve before her severed sister Ereshkigal swallows her whole with pain, grief, and anger.

My explorations in witchcraft brought freedom: it was a massive part of my waxing toward becoming the Maiden. It felt like no one in our mainstream culture was coming out as a witch yet, nobody in the mainstream was talking about the Goddess—especially not anyone in my very normal company. Witches were made fun of; they were just something you dressed up as for Halloween, or as we witches call it, Samhain. But I felt an internal power when I used my spell books, when I created altars, and then again when I went into the woods for healing rituals. Eventually I could go off-script and leave the manuals behind as my intuition grew and I could feel my way into what the right incantation was for the moment.

When I initially reclaimed witch, it was intense work of de-stigmatization, over and over again. People would say things to me like, "Oh congratulations, do you drink people's blood? Do you sacrifice animals? Do you work with the devil?"

Everything I shared online about "witch" went viral. Women expressed so much glee over it, and it started to spread like crazy. I soon was convinced that every woman was a witch; we'd just all forgotten it. "Witch" as an archetype represents what it means to be an ancient feminine Goddess before a culture that demonized the Goddess had stolen our earthly, seasonal realities and rituals.

It became the work of making it something beautiful again, of taking it from the profane back to the sacred. It was a deep reclamation of something taken from us, and my life has never been the same. Eventually, you stop practicing so much magic and just become it.

It was fun to help women with spells and share all the magic books I was reading. Finding out that my mother had her own secrets related to witchcraft gave me even more insight into my path. Receiving the box with her runes and spell books that she had kept hidden helped me understand that when women hide their witch, they're repressing their natural power, their natural path to the wise woman and healer. I held my first witch circle in 2011, which nobody I knew was doing at the time. I started to teach women how to hold these circles; I'd write about it on my website to disseminate the remembrance.

When I began to do this work, it had a powerful effect because the power of women coming together with the same intention to heal themselves, each other, and the Earth can't be overstated: it is the reason covens were disbanded and made illegal. Women I was connected to started to hold these literal circles all over the world. They were women sitting in a hoop around a central altar, sharing their truths.

Why circles? Because they abolish the hierarchy of the old paradigm way of teaching, where one person holds the power and everyone else is subordinate as the power is outside of them, in the teacher. Just as we learn to re-mother ourselves in this work, we also re-educate. Many of the women I work with were too sensitive for the schooling systems they were placed in as children. They were taught to be subservient and to conform. There was trauma for the disciplinarian way they were taught. I was often sent out of class or to the principal for my daydreaming, for my questioning the teacher.

But there are no grades in feminine wisdom, no hierarchical order, no passing or failing or punishment and discipline. The Maiden is safe to express herself and to question everything.

They also bring us back to our source because circles are a fundamental organizing formation in nature. The sun and moon rise and set in a circle around the sphere of the Earth. The year's seasons form a great circle. Whirling everywhere is the spiral wind, which carries the birds, who make their nests in circles.

These rituals of holding space for one another, grounding ourselves in the earth, and drawing boundaries around how much we could give help us restore our energy so we can contribute more appropriately and become whole. As a group, we model mature feminine friendships and show each other compassion, while listening with open hearts. Our connection is based on common pains and a shared longing to move through it without destruction. We reject the fairy tales that have given us the negative witch image, and together we create the positive.

In the story of Inanna, there's a character named Ninshubar, who is Inanna's closest counsel. She's the healer a woman needs to hold space for her as she descends to her severed self. Before Inanna goes, she says, "If I'm not back in three days, send to the fathers for help." Ninshubar keeps watch from above. She's there if and when Inanna needs her.

It's imperative to recognize that we need help on this journey. I always advise women to work with a therapist or healer who has access to soul and archetypal language on this part of the journey.

It's important that you have someone you trust to keep the spelunking rope connected to you when you journey into the dark of your repressed psyche. You go down alone, supported by a midwife or coven overhead, tracking and rooting for your rebirth.

When we first meet the pain we have ignored for the first act of our life, it can feel like it's killing us. Had Inanna not told Ninshubar to send for help, she'd never have made it back to life. When Inanna does not return after three days, Ninshubar knows to get help. (Sidenote: We'd all go to the underworld and collect our lost selves if we could just schedule it for a long weekend, but the three days are symbolic in this myth, representing life, death, rebirth. Alas, it takes as long as it takes in the underworld.)

When Ninshubar runs to the two fathers, Enil and Nanna, both refuse to help the Goddess. They reason that she has broken their rules, and this is her punishment. Inanna knew that only when we break the rules that are killing us do we stand a chance at survival. Well-behaved women rarely make history, as the saying goes.

But this is a moment of cold, cruel awakening, for the reader of this myth, and for Inanna: we are only protected when we play by the rules, when we are good, when we do as they say, when we are the nice little girl. Our protection is conditional upon our submission to authority.

Ninshubar then goes to Father Enki, the God of Water. A man of balanced masculine and feminine energies, he feels and grieves for Inanna. He carves two sexless flies, or "demons," from the clay beneath his nails and sends them to retrieve Inanna from the underworld. They fly down to the belly of the underworld, and they attend to Ereshkigal. They hover over her in vigil. The concept of demon is very important here. Demons symbolize what we are afraid of in ourselves and in the world, and they must be faced head-on to achieve liberation. When we confront them, we learn to listen to our inner selves.

Held by the vigil of these flies, Ereshkigal explodes with grief. Her husband is dead, and now she has killed her sister. She begins to moan, like a woman caught between life and death. Her cries are not quite of grief and not quite of birth. Something in between.

Ereshkigal stands in for the most dangerous and dark pieces of our inner world, lying naked on the ground, grieving, and having killed. The fly demons see her at her absolute worst, and instead of rejecting her, they softly, empathetically ask her what ails her. They mirror her without judgment, without any attempts to fix her or tell her what to do. I imagine that their dialogue went something like this:

"What ails you?" they ask.

"I'm sad," she says.

"You're sad," they say.

She hears herself.

"Why are you sad?"

"My husband died, and then I killed my sister."

"Your husband died, and then you killed your sister."

"Yes."

"Why did you kill your sister?"

"Because I was angry."

"You were angry."

"I missed her."

"You missed her."

"I've been down here all along, all alone, all this time."

"You've been down here all along, all alone, all this time."

"It's so lonely."

"It's so lonely."

"I'm afraid."

"You're afraid."

"I want to be seen."

"You want to be seen."

"I want to be heard."

"You want to be heard."

"I want to be held."

"You want to be held."

This compassionate exchange of active listening, but not fixing—the act of not saving someone so that they can save themselves—holds up a mirror so a woman can see herself. The repetition of her words offers a woman space to hear herself. Our work is to see our true selves and to listen to our true selves. When the little flies dare to approach this heaving, grieving mess of a woman at her worst, they exhibit the courage and compassion necessary for her transformation.

When she rises, she ascends with remembrance, acceptance, and purpose.

Reflection Exercise: Compassionately Listening to Your Maiden

In this exercise, we will go deep inside to where your Maiden dwells and listen actively and compassionately to her feelings. This gives her the space to grow in ways she hasn't been able to, previously. Begin by closing your eyes and taking deep, slow breaths. Root deeply into whatever holds your body, knowing whatever chair, bed, or floor you're on eventually connects to the Earth, to the Great Mother, to the body of the Goddess.

Feel that reunion. Feel yourself being held. Feel the release and relief of letting go.

Imagine the air around you is full of cherishing Mother energy that celebrates every single shadow, every dusty nook and cranny of you. Imagine the air is thick with swirling energy and start to drink it like a thirsty child.

Inside of you, your inner Maiden is being fed, being served that loving Mother energy. Let her drink it up and feel full of love for herself so she has it to give to others. Let the place where you are sitting or lying hold you. This is your time to practice being held. Whatever you rest upon connects to the Great Mother—the Great Mother that longs to have her children return to her. Feel her pulsing and breathing in your body as your body becomes soft and receptive, opening as much as possible to the wisdom that awaits you.

As you slow your breath, imagine your most beloved place in nature: a place you feel safe, warm, and relaxed. This might be a beach, jungle, forest, desert, or another place near and dear to you. Let yourself fully arrive, taking in the serene and beautiful landscape. Notice how good it feels to be there. Imagine now seeing a cave in this beautiful place. This cave is safe, secluded, and also a part of sacred Earth herself.

Feel the strength of your own body. The energy inside, waiting, ready, and vigilant to protect and nurture. Then with your Mother presence, scan around inside. When we come in to witness the inner Maiden, we come in as Mother.

Tell those parts of you:
"I'm right here.
I love you.
I see you.
I hear you.
And I'm not going anywhere.
You have my word.
And even if my word hasn't been much until now, from every day forward you have my word.
And I will prove my love to you. I'm home now."

As your body becomes the cave itself, notice there is an opening at the top. Approach it, knowing how safe you are. Slowly begin to enter the cave of your body. Take your time, and spiral down, down, down to the very bottom of the cave. Notice the muddy, dirty floor here. Notice what the bottom of the cave looks like and feels like.

Begin to sense that there is someone down there waiting for you. This is the little you, your Maiden. Some of the women I work with have found it helpful to prepare for this exercise by looking at childhood photos. As your maiden begins to show herself to you, keep your body language open and compassionate, and give her plenty of space as you stay on your side of the cave (giving her room is especially important if this is your first meeting). Take your time locating her and observing her, don't rush or force anything, and always trust your experience.

Take notice of her details. What are your first impressions of her? What is her approximate age? What is she wearing? One of my clients found her maiden totally disheveled, wearing rags, and whimpering. If she's been down there for a long time all by herself, feeling abandoned or neglected, that might be the case. Or she might be clean and well taken care of. However she appears, observe her with your highest, most compassionate self from the perspective of a cherishing Mother.

Notice what she's doing. Is she touching or holding anything? Eating or playing? Crying? Is she hiding from you or crawling all over you? What's her body language like? Is she sitting, standing, lying down? How does she seem? What is her emotion or mood? Sad, scared, playful? Trust whatever she shows you and know that here there is no right or wrong.

Staying on your side of the cave, give her space as you watch on with gentle, loving eyes. Say hello to her softly. She may speak to you back, and she might not. She might be angry, anxious, worried, afraid, or happy to see you. Now say to her: How are you? As she responds, practice simple reflexive listening with her.

She might say, I'm sad. You then softly respond: Why are you sad? A few other examples might be:

I'm angry. Why are you angry?

I'm lonely. Why are you lonely?

I'm afraid. Why are you afraid?

I'm happy. Why are you happy?

As she responds, keep reflecting back to her with compassion.

She might say: I'm lonely/angry/sad because you haven't visited me. You would then say: Why haven't I visited you? Listen to her and keep responding with compassion.

For example, she might then say: Because you have had to be an adult. You then respond: Why did it make you lonely/sad/ angry that I had to be an adult?

Continue interacting with her as you reflect back her experience. Give her your full attention as you engage in this safe dialogue. Take your time interacting with her and getting to know her feelings and perspective.

Then ask her:

What can I do to make you feel safe? Seen? Loved?

What do you need from me, right now in this moment?

What can I do for you?

Stay with her and continue to spend time with her, as you may now want to come closer to one another. She may want to play, or color, or have some tea. She may have another request of you, such as making a boundary in your life. She might ask for you to visit every day. She simply might want to be held or have you sing her a song. A song she may like is: I love you, I'm right here, I'm not going anywhere.

There will be internal and external requests. Our work on this relationship between Maiden and Mother—in order to create that stable attachment again (or maybe for the first time ever)—is to follow up on what we promise we will do. This helps build trust again. Tell her you are here for her and love her.

As your interaction comes to a close, tell her you will come back. Explain to her that you have to go, but that you are listening to her and that she can call on you when she needs you. Tell her you will hear her and honor her.

Then, say goodbye to her.

Start to rise through your cave, up through the spiral staircase, up, up, up, close the door to the cave. Bow to the cave, the cave of your body where your Maiden rests. Come back into your resting place and slowly open your eyes and return to your surroundings. When you feel ready, wiggle your toes and fingers, and feel the sensation of cherishing Mother energy pouring into you. Slowly and gently come back to your body and into your space.

Now journal your experience.

JOURNAL PROMPTS

How do you feel? What did this exercise bring up for you?

What does it feel like to tend yourself with the cherishing Mother energy of unconditional love?

What do you notice about how you feel in this moment versus how you felt before this exercise?

What did you notice about your Maiden? What was her age? What was she wearing? How did she seem?

Did you receive any request(s)? If so, how will you begin to tend to whatever it is your inner self is asking you for?

What have you learned from her about how to be her Mother?

THREE-MINUTE MAIDEN CHECK-IN

After you have formally met your Maiden through the Maiden meditation, it is essential to check in on your Maiden regularly, just the way a parent would check in with a child. It can be helpful to establish a daily check-in where the two of you spend, say, three minutes together. When your

Maiden is attended to and cared for, you will be amazed at how your life changes.

Find a quiet place where you will be uninterrupted. Take three big breaths and exhale through your mouth and come into your body, the belly of you. Imagine the air around you is full of cherishing Mother energy and drink it in again.

When you feel ready, whisper to your Maiden: I'm here with you. I love you. I'm checking in on you. Feel her arriving. Don't worry if this doesn't happen right away. With practice, she will start to become more familiar. Then whisper to your Maiden: How are you? What do you need?

Listen to her response with compassion. If she is feeling shy and not ready to speak, give her time and space to open up. She may have a lot to say or speak only a few words.

Tell her you will get her what she needs to be her best. Tell her you'll see her tomorrow. Slowly open your eyes and come back to the room.

VISITING YOUR MAIDEN SEASONALLY

You may also be excited to connect more with the Earth in the spirit of our witch women ancestors. I, personally, have been drawn to celebrating the solstices and equinoxes, when the Earth is in a powerful, transformative position in relation to the sun, four times each year. You might choose to honor this passage around the sun, which symbolizes death and rebirth, by visiting your maiden at these points in the year. As the Earth shifts seasonally, so do we. In fall and winter, all living beings turn inward, and we are pulled to do the same. As spring brings rebirth, we are moved to rise back up toward the sun and offer our gifts again. In summer we burn bright, in autumn we fall back to the Earth, in winter we go dormant, and so on. We celebrate and stay aligned with the seasonal shifts Mother Earth is moving through, and that we, as natural beings, are moving through too. Tap into how your Maiden heals at these times for a powerful practice to help you track her growth.

TROUBLESHOOTING
THE MAIDEN MEDITATION

1. Trust your first inner visions. Overthinking this exercise does not serve you or allow an authentic experience to arise. Let the images come to you and trust them.

2. No judging, fixing, or explaining to your Maiden, just curiosity and witnessing her. Let her lead and reveal herself to you.

3. If you feel you are leaving your Maiden when she is not in a good place—don't worry, this means you just need to come back regularly and visit her. Over time she will become more nourished and increasingly less abandoned when you need to leave.

4. If your encounter is overwhelming to you—don't push yourself. Go slow and maybe return to this meditation on a day you feel more ready. Also, consider doing the meditation in small doses versus all of it at once.

5. Know that your Maiden may appear at any age and any stage of your life. Often she is a little girl. Sometimes she's a teenager, sometimes older or younger.

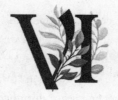

Becoming a Medicine Woman

Don't be that wounded healer
Who can heal everyone
but herself.
Don't be that medicine woman
who serves everyone else
while her own dose
Remains on the shelf.

After Inanna descends through the seven gates to meet face-to-face the severed parts of herself, her furious, scorned, and abandoned sister, Ereshkigal, kills her. This rabid woman has been down in the underworld all alone with Inanna's pain, the gory, human pain that wasn't permissible in the upperworld. She's been holding it all for Inanna. It's heavy. It's lonely. It's killing her.

By the time she sees that the beautiful and light Inanna has deigned to visit her in the basement of the world, Ereshkigal is boiling over. She is terrified, heartbroken, and enraged. After the murder, she hangs Inanna on a meat hook, where she begins to rot.

The moment we face our darkness kills us temporarily; it is the reason why we get so nervous when we express the intention to claim lost parts of ourselves. It's scary when you say, "I'm going to face what I've been running from. I'm ready to heal," because healing will mean irrevocably changing your life. Healing will kill what is killing you. The battle looms, which means a warrior, or heroine, will have to be born.

The first time you say, "I'm going to leap off this known shore for the unknown depths, for a call I cannot explain," everyone balks. You might hear: "Don't do that. Don't face your darkness. It will kill you." And it will. The false, small parts of you will die. You will be on your way to becoming authentic and whole.

You will come back with the dark parts of you. You will come back with your power.

So here is the corpse of Inanna, slain by her sister Ereshkigal. The little flies had just actively listened to Ereshkigal, which allowed her to feel heard, to feel held, and therefore to begin the process to heal. In response to such a compassionate healing experience, Ereshkigal asks the flies what she can do for them in return. They'd like the corpse of Inanna, they say, and their request is granted (with a catch—but we'll get to that later).

The flies then sprinkle the bread and water of life onto Inanna's corpse, and she slowly comes back to life. She gingerly rises like a newborn foal, on wobbly legs, with new eyes to see, a cleansed heart, a strengthened soul, a renewed sense of purpose.

Inanna knew this day would come and she would be reborn. As she was a priestess of Earth, she was aligned with the cycles of nature deeply and intimately. She knew that after the death of winter comes the bloom of spring. This is how she had the courage to say yes to the call of the underworld, even though everybody told her not to go.

On her ascent back up from the underworld, Inanna healed one chakra at every gate she passed through, starting with her root chakra. At the first gate, her roots to the Earth were restored. Then, her sensuality at her second chakra was returned. Next, her solar plexus was restored, and her purpose clarified. Her fourth chakra—her heart—was healed from past pain and threw open its golden gates. Her fifth chakra—her throat—was cleared, and her voice was reclaimed. At her third eye, she claimed the seat of witness: she would no longer be the reactive little girl but the responsive woman. She was responsible for her power. And finally at her crown chakra, her divinity and queenlike inner royalty was cemented. She returned as the priestess of Heaven and Earth.

But, as with all changes and all portals we move through, something must be lost for everything gained. Inanna had to leave her wounded Maiden life in the underworld in exchange for the archetypal Mother life she rose into. Part of herself died for this new life.

While Inanna journeys to the underworld just once, I've found that a non-mythical life is far messier, with lessons that may take a long time to sink in fully. Fighting your way out of the darkness once does not guarantee that you will stay in the light thereafter. Women especially are cyclical. We wax and wane, shifting in response to the natural world, our internal compass, and circumstances in our lives. We may waiver in our certainty and poise, slipping out of Mother and back into Maiden again. It is very common to visit the underworld multiple times over the course of your life. Yet each time you do, you gain more of yourself back, and you gain more tools and wisdom to navigate this fertile rebirth territory.

Three years after my awakening to the Goddess, I found myself descending again. Directly behind my heart, a tick with

Lyme disease had embedded into my back, injecting me with its destructive program. By the time I had discovered it, I was trapped for days in winter's worst snowstorm. I couldn't do anything to prevent the ensuing fatigue and pain that would plague me for years. Struggling against this illness, I threw myself into every kind of treatment and possible cure. I liked to say that I was trying to get the weight of one thousand elephants off my chest. My symptoms would advance and recede, but nothing I tried could ever stop the elephant from settling in again. I was getting desperate for relief, and I slid into a depression. Yet my work with women on their spiritual journeys was what kept me going during this period of exhaustion, and my practice really began to grow, which allowed me to spend more resources on my health.

I had a simple prayer at the time. It was to become my own medicine woman. It stemmed from my urge to stop—ever again—seeking someone to tell me how to live or what to do or how to help or how to heal myself. Remember the Jungian analyst Marie-Louise von Franz, who discussed how becoming a medicine woman begins by falling into the power of the demons? She said that when you wrench yourself up from the deep, dark space, you are initiated into your medicine power, the power of Mother.

As a woman transforms into Mother, she cares for all her wounded, unloved, unseen, unheld, unheard—and therefore unhealed—places. When a woman comes into Mother, she becomes a medicine woman because the Mother is the medicine she needs and the Mother is the medicine the world needs. My prayer and intention to become my own medicine woman suddenly led to signs from the intelligence beyond my own head. I began to follow these signs, perhaps a little too far.

One dark day as I was struggling to get my slow-as-molasses body up the stairs, I leaned heavily on the railing, and the lyrics of a song I vaguely knew flew into my head.

"The pain that comes today/

Is here, then goes away/

And we are homeward bound/

And I . . . I want this more than life."[14]

I remembered it was sung by this boyishly cute, dark-haired, and sullen indie rocker, Whitley, who had talked about his experiences with depression and how the plant medicine ayahuasca had helped him. It was as if my memory of him had been unearthed by my inner Mother. I could feel a pull from where my umbilical cord was, like she was pulling me toward this medicine. I started to read about this ancient cure, made from a powerful vine and an activating plant by pre-colonial South American healing shamans. Its psychedelic properties induced ego-shattering visions that were alleged to cure a range of ailments, including inflammatory diseases like Lyme. I was suddenly curious if my path led to ayahuasca. But how would I find it?

Then I connected a few more dots to my future path. A month prior, a psychic astrologer I visited to seek answers about my condition had told me that I was born to be a medicine woman. This didn't sound right to me. How could I be a healer when I was so damaged? But I trusted that there was a message there. As I searched for a way to be initiated, I sought counsel from my recently deceased aunt Lisa who had been killed by a car in her prime. She was the first woman in our family to be openly spiritual, the first woman I knew who openly expressed the power of her inner witch, and I had looked up to her immensely. Lisa had done her work; she had done the descent and the rebirth and the rise and the offering of her soul as a gift. She had gifted me a short memoir about a woman's spiritual awakening, but I was keeping it to read for a special time. I knew that if anyone would have something to say to me about ayahuasca, it would be her. As I grabbed the memoir from my shelf, it fell open to a page with this line: "I spent the winter solstice (December 21) in Peru."

I felt hopeful for the first time in many months. This message of synchronicity was Mother telling me exactly how to find my medicine. I searched online and found a Peruvian ayahuasca center that called to me. I was terrified of this voyage to the unknown but driven to discover my way out of the underworld again.

Before my fear could talk me down, I bought a session at the retreat during my birthday and the winter solstice, plus a plane ticket. I knew it was probably naive of me to rush head-long into this unknown world. I wasn't used to international travel, I didn't speak any Spanish, and I had a vague sense that I didn't quite understand what I might encounter as a white, privileged Westerner seeking out potent indigenous wisdom.

I tried to stay focused on the strong signs and messages I had received pointing me toward this trip. A friend told me that there's never a good time for ayahuasca. There's no convenient moment for your life as you know it to change completely. It's got to be an abrupt decision: you're always too busy—and that's the point. That's why you need to change your life. My resistance to the trip quickly transformed into childish glee and anticipation. I got caught up in the potential for metamorphosis, and my inner Maiden rose inside of me. I started to see the trip as a chance for a romantic adventure, not acknowledging that I was still ill and suffering from a deep heart-wound, one that went back decades, and was further entrenched by that tick.

But I leaped. I flew to Peru. Once inside a new country, out of my comfort zone, I was scared, as it became clear that I was grossly unprepared for life outside the castle. Perpetually tripping over my long, flowing dress, I struggled like a pack mule under five different bags so stuffed that they couldn't even zip up properly. As a bumbling gringo, I relied on hand gestures, signs, and goodwill to find my way to the center. When I made it to that mountaintop retreat, I fell sick from the altitude. My breath grew shallow with a debilitating headache, and the cramps of my impending period felt like daggers repeatedly thrust into my womb. Yet I tried to push away these symptoms, attempting to focus on the green, rolling hills outside my window that framed an enchanted storybook land of handcrafted cottages. I believed I was in the fairy tale I had waited for since childhood.

That first night, I had dinner alone, and I tuned in to the guests' chatter about the owner, who was also the shaman. My antenna picked up; I was so curious about who would be serving us medicine, but I couldn't make out what they were saying.

I'd meet him soon enough in the first ceremony, in a big white yurt lit up at night. The shaman walked in late to address our group, which I'd come to understand was his way of hooking participants into his magnetic orbit. I'd get to know him very, very personally. But at this first impression, he was formidable, handsome, and mysterious. I thought I was in a spiritual meet-cute with this well-built British man with piercing blue eyes and long, thick black hair. After introducing us to the ritual of ayahuasca, he knelt in front of me with massive hands holding out the cup of magical elixir. That first drink experience was an ecstatic return to the Goddess—I felt cherishing Mother love and a sense of unity and peace about all the time

I had spent in the underworld. Among many visions of strange tropical vistas crawling with creatures I'd never encountered, I also saw the shaman implanting my womb with a radiant golden egg. When I came down, I convinced myself that this was just an immature interpretation of my developing crush on the shaman. It couldn't mean anything else.

Then came the second ayahuasca ceremony, when he began to work one-on-one with me, helping me release my lingering heartaches, for Tim, for my mother, and for all the time I had spent not knowing who I was. I was vulnerable and raw with him, which he insisted upon, as he blew pipe smoke into my belly button, chanting in a language I had never heard. I felt a flicker of recognition that the attraction was brewing.

That night, he walked me out of the ceremony and lingered outside my door as if we'd been on a great first date. I had heard he never went to clients' rooms except when working privately with them in isolation (for a large fee). But here he was at mine, asking me if I needed anything, if my room was warm enough, if I knew how to properly load my wood stove.

"Yes," I said hesitantly, "everything is fine."

I smiled politely. I was aware of my past drama patterns with dynamic, commanding men and felt my inner Mother pulling me back inside to protect me. He said goodbye and closed the door.

And suddenly I knew: "He's going to knock again."

Bang, bang.

"Yes?"

"I think we should talk about the feelings I have for you."

And that was when I pushed back against my inner Mother, that strong sense of self-love that I had deliberately cultivated over years that had driven me to seek the medicine so I could come into full bloom. I turned away from that nourishing, centered source, and allowed my Maiden, fresh with lust and the desire to be desired, still bleeding from past wounds that she had only loosely bandaged, to fully claim the room, which suddenly became a portal back to the underworld.

What followed was his seduction of me that night—the unethical entrapment of a client and guest who'd laid her life's pain at his feet. He knew all my wounds from the retreat center intake form, and he used his understanding of my psyche to get what he wanted. His energy was electrically attractive, and I couldn't pull away.

My Maiden believed that he knew what was best for me and that I needed to take his medicine, his wisdom, and his instruction to expel the darkness within me. The Mother in me had intended to come to the brief retreat for the initiation into ayahuasca to heal my Lyme disease and learn the power of plant medicine. Still, I ended up staying for months at a time, returning to my home only to check on my former life and then running back into the nest he and I were creating in his magnificent mountaintop cottage. We had a spiritual community supporting us, fascinating people to connect with and to explore the landscape with, and a staff that cooked us meals and cleaned our home. But I knew that we were getting snared in an unhealthy, sometimes psychotic, relationship fueled by drugs and manipulation.

One time, he demanded that I remain in a room by myself for a week, drinking tobacco three times a day until I threw up. He told me to read books to change my thinking about the dark feminine, and he would come in periodically and ask if I agreed with his understanding that there was something wrong with me and it was up to him to fix me. And when I'd resist, he'd rise from the chair coldly and tell me I needed more time alone. When I begged to leave, he said that if I did, he'd break up with me and I'd have to make it down the mountain, through rural towns, and back to Lima by myself. One day during that isolation, weak and disoriented, I looked out the window to see a white wolf. She stared directly into my eyes and then moved away.

I told him I'd seen her. The Mother.

"There are no wolves in Peru," he said, completely dismissing my intuition.

He used the ayahuasca medicine to change me from wild to subservient. Over those months, I slowly realized I was tied to an insane person, though the specific diagnosis eluded me. Sometimes I would realize that I was once again prisoner of a hypnotic, patriarchal fairy tale. But I had more moments when I truly believed he was my rescuer. It was the inverse of *Beauty and the Beast.* Instead of being trapped in a castle with a beast who turns into a prince, I was trapped with a prince who turned into a beast.

My mother wound opened further, and I felt once again acutely that my mother had never loved me, which meant I could never be loved. Like the moment when I promised to hate myself after she died, I felt like I deserved him. Being with this destructive man demonstrated how much I really did hate myself. Utterly exhausted and beaten, I resigned myself to a life with him. Because at the same time he imprisoned me, he also offered me opportunities to expand my work, to bring people inspired by my work to the center to partake of ayahuasca and change their lives for the better.

Then, I got pregnant.

I recalled my vision of the golden egg on my first night at the retreat center. This symbol was a portal to my future, though I had scoffed at its importance on my first night with ayahuasca. This egg was now inside of me. And with that new life growing, my wounded Maiden spell was broken. I finally heard Goddess, the Mother, calling to me through nightmares, inner alarms, and wolf howls. It became clear: I had to leave. Otherwise, I would be crushed under his weight. I was still no good at saving myself, but I would save the baby. Or perhaps it was saving me?

Our culture trains us to wait in a pretty dress for masculine saviors. The damsel-in-distress myth damns us. It tricks us into believing we are fragile, and it programs us to be fearful little girls in women's bodies. Through media and cultural messages, we are continuously coached to be desirable to men by staying forever young and disempowered. When whittled down to their core message, these fairytales say: WAIT. STAY. Wait, trapped under glass like Snow White. Stay sleeping until the prince comes. Wait in the tower of your life while it's under attack; stay for the one who is coming.

Maybe a savior would arrive, but often he was a man dominated by the immature masculine, who poses as a rescuer before he reveals that he is really a petulant child, or far worse: a captor, abuser, or villain.

In Maiden, we refuse to listen to our intuition, our inner Mother. The Maiden is always in a rush to satisfy herself and others, while the Mother is very slow. Maiden reaches out to others for the things she can't yet access within: love, validation, and comfort. In Maiden, we go looking to men to parent us instead of partner with us. We do not have access to our needs, and therefore, we are unable to speak them clearly, which leads to resentment, tantrums, and reactive drama. We say things like, "I couldn't help myself," or "I couldn't control myself." We incite jealousy to make him want us more, and we compete with other women for his attention. This all comes from deep insecurity.

When I became pregnant by my abuser, I couldn't play small anymore if I wanted to survive. In a flash of insight, I called upon the Mother's compassionate love. I'd need to navigate every decision now as if I loved myself.

I would have to finally face the fear he brought up in me: that I was helpless and unsafe. I would not be able to rest until I learned to fight for myself. I was going to have to wake up and deal with the threat. Like a rose, I needed to root and rise, and find my sword-like thorns. I had gotten myself into this compromised situation, and I was going to have to get myself out of it. I was being asked to stand up for myself and claim my worth. The circumstances demanded I claim my power or die.

They raised you to be the princess
They took away your right to fight
only the fearless know what I mean
when you die to the princess and rise to the queen
when you descend to the depths to begin again
when you die to rise whole
when you lose everything
but in your soul, you're no longer a Maiden; you're the Mother
you possess a power like no other
don't stay sleeping under the glass case
don't run from the dragon
face your face
don't stay trapped in your terrified tower
this is your moment, this is your hour,
you are the queen of the night

And also the brave knight
and this is your life
And this is your fight

I don't remember much about how I left, but when I landed in the airport back at home, I knew I still wasn't safe. I'd gotten physically away from the shaman, but he had been harassing and threatening me online, lying about me, and calling my phone only to say something haunting and hang up. I didn't know where he was; this phantom who could strike at any moment. But I had Ereshkigal and all the buried dark feminine power that was unearthed in my descent to meet myself. The Goddess and her infinite expressions are as fierce as they are beautiful.

Heavily pregnant, I began seeing an acupuncturist and friend named Cathleen. She was a calm and confident healer, a mature and beautiful woman who took sublime care of herself so she could take sublime care of others. She was an archetypal Mother. One day, I lay before this medicine woman, crying on the table beneath her needles.

"What's he like?" Cathleen asked me tenderly.

"You know Jimmy Angelov? Nicole Kidman's ex in the film *Practical Magic*?" I said. "The one that dies and comes back to life, and they have to call a coven of housewives from the school phone tree to exorcise him from the house? That's him."

She laughed through her worried expression. "At least you still have your sense of humor."

And it's true; I knew how to laugh even amid the terror, at least for a moment. There were small windows between gusts of reality where I could pretend the terror wasn't happening. That's how I used to survive. Pretending is a coping survival mechanism. I could pretend it wasn't happening.

That day on the acupuncturist's healing table, I wanted Cathleen to feel sorry for me and say, "I'll help you." But she did better than that. She said, "It's time for you to fight your own battles." There was no one else left to reach for to protect me and fight *for* me.

When I first begin working with some women on their Maiden-to-Mother journey, their initial inclination is to reach for me to save them. They project what they needed from their own mother onto me. There is a smallness and helplessness in them that hopes I'll take care of them. But I can't do that. It wouldn't serve them; it would only put a bandage on their gaping Maiden wounds. Save a woman in the moment, and it saves her for the day. Teach her to save herself, and it saves her for a lifetime. Cathleen knew that.

I simply didn't know how to save myself before. I didn't have the tools because they weren't taught to or shown to me, because they aren't taught or shown to girls in this society.

The day Cathleen told me it was time to fight for myself was the day I picked up my sword and began to swashbuckle my way out of the tower I'd waited in since I was a child. That was the day I decided I was worthy of protection. I called the local domestic shelter and started the process of getting a restraining order against my baby's father.

My reference to *Practical Magic* wasn't just funny; it was true. This work is not unlike an exorcism, healing the toxic masculine and patriarchy out of the bodies and souls of women. There's a place in my process of Maiden-to-Mother teachings where I stop acknowledging the wounded Maiden in the woman at all. I refuse to feed the patriarchalized feminine in her; I starve it by not responding to it. If she complains about someone else or expresses self-pity, I tell her to try again. I choose to only see and respond to the Mother in her. And that Mother rises, getting stronger with each acknowledgment. She is the one who heals the little girl within.

When I taught my online Maiden-to-Mother journeys, I'd speak to a coven of women, dozens of them all somewhere out there in the dark. I told my own stories of rebirth and wove them with Goddess Inanna's descent and reclaiming herself.

The power of a women's circle can't be overstated. The medicine of others witnessing you telling your story of darkness, the medicine of hearing your tale spill from another woman's mouth, is liberating because it's so de-isolating. I-solating kills. We-llness heals.

Before that circle, you might think you're alone. You're conditioned to keep your scary, strange secrets to yourself because we've been told we must conform to the ideal of a good girl. The simple, but previously banished, act of women coming together erases this messaging. Women communicating and supporting one another in sisterhood is a direct threat to the patriarchy and its rules for women and girls. Historically, covens were banished for fear of the power of a group of women holding the same intention together and fear of the empowerment bestowed on women in sisterhood. A miracle occurs when you hear your most terrifying story or feelings bubble from the cauldron of someone else. For the same reason, the #MeToo movement is wildly liberating, which is to say, healing. Women telling their stories is not intended for men primarily. It is for that other woman out there, huddled in her closet, to hear. It is for her to say: "Me, too," and to leave her dark cave and tell her story for another woman who will be able to say, "Me, too." We need the dark feminine to become whole; it gives us our teeth and our tears, our full range of emotions and humanity, our authenticity, and our realness. The dark feminine empowers us to take up the sword of the Mother.

I first brandished my sword in the courtroom, telling the judge why I deserved to be protected. And I won. Other women brandish their swords when they acknowledge how their fathers abandoned or abused them, how lovers stole their innocence, how employers denigrated them, or how strangers objectified them. When they walk out, talk back, and build a wall around themselves, they are taking up their swords.

The feminist poet Adrienne Rich has written about powerful moments of self-protection. "Sometimes this involves tiny acts of immense courage; sometimes public acts which can cost a woman her job or her life; often it involves moments, or long periods, of thinking the unthinkable, being labeled, or feeling crazy; [it's] always a loss of traditional securities."[15]

Rich expressed hope for the women who do this, and also for the men who witness it. A woman understands that by taking her life in her own hands, she may experience enormous pain, internally and externally. Rich sees women as better able to face this pain, perhaps born from our position as the life-givers and those who birth with extreme discomfort. Men must learn not to shrink from this pain, wherever it occurs. Unearthing their dark stories is part of bringing light to the world and disinfecting us from the patriarchy.

I know the power of story. Secret-keeping is imprisonment, but secret-releasing is liberation. Story by story, the patriarchy falls like dominos. One story nudges the next, and that one knocks at the next, until the whole prison falls to that holy ground, where we can begin again.

And our stories heal each other. For women, when you hear another woman's story and you feel your compassion for her, you realize you can apply that to yourself. You hear yourself think, *That's not so scary; she'll be okay*, and then you realize you can also apply *that* to yourself. You get to realize, once again, you're not alone. We all have the same fears: terror of being seen, terror of not being seen, and a fear of being exiled. We contain the deep desire to use our true voices, yet we struggle with the terror of rejection.

Girls who don't experience feminine rites of passage into the powerful and mature feminine have relied instead on men, and masculine gods and governments, who had no interest in helping or saving them, to show them how to behave. We follow their rules until their rules kill us. We hide to survive until the hiding that saved us starves us. This cycle continues until finally, finally, one princess picks up the sword, saves herself, and becomes the queen.

Furthermore, the men who perpetrate abuse must become accountable. Their actions have deeply damaged humanity, silencing women who might have been powerful examples of the full feminine. Instead, these survivors are forced to spend years, sometimes their whole lifetimes, seeking healing and reintegration. Yet, our culture has yet to recognize that the men are also seeking the same thing. As bell hooks wrote, "The first act of violence that patriarchy demands of males is not violence toward women. Instead, patriarchy demands of all males that they engage in acts of psychic self-mutilation; it asks that they kill off the emotional parts of themselves."[16]

Just as the feminine rites of passage were buried, the rite of passage from boy to man, or prince to king, is missing from our culture. And just like women, men suffer greatly without these rites of passage. When earth religions centered on rites of passage and seasonal alignment were vilified, the kings and queens died. Men stayed boys. Women stayed girls to the detriment of the entire world.

Now, women feel like they're doing all the work to heal. This question comes up all the time: What about the men? They need this passage too. Angry, abused, and therefore abusive boys in men's bodies, suffering from lack of the Mother (and the true, healed Father), are everywhere. When I mention healthy masculinity in my teachings, women ask, "What is that? We don't have a model for that."

At the Rites of Passage Institute, leader and teacher Kamya O'Keeffe works to initiate boys into maturity. For most men, this rite of passage involves creating a deep space for emotional vulnerability. This is something men don't have in a culture that encourages them to be bullies and be at war. They come into circle (which is by nature feminine, if you consider the moon, the Earth, and the womb). With elders, who model the healthy, mature masculine, the boys (or men still living as boys) are encouraged to feel, share, open, and offer their insecurities and fears. This is transformative for many of them because they feel like they have to be so tough in the outer world. Then, there is time spent in nature, where they are asked to begin to honor the feminine, Mother Nature, and Mother energy. It's a small vision quest for "What sort of man do you want to be?" It creates a model and map.

I have learned to remember, inside of me, the sacred masculine. I have recalled the lover, the healer, the good man, the warrior, the wizard, the poet, the soulful, divine masculine man who stays and protects, feels, cries, shares, and openly loves. It wasn't until I could remember him on the inside that I would see him again on the outside. The Maiden only recognizes the boy, but Mother can see the man.

When you have seen a woman claim her sword, and her Goddess power, you know that you can only be matched by a man as brave as you are. This is an initiated man, who embodies heart-centered masculinity. He's a man who has braved his hero's journey, inwardly. The descent to the Goddess, whose love they haven't fully experienced. Men in our culture are taught to conquer, claim, compete, dominate, and win. They spend their lives accumulating money and goods that symbolize their conquests. In the vision of the warrior, there is no space for vulnerability and compassion. Yet if they could explore their own terrifying underworlds, they could bring back a healed man who can give himself in humble, strong service to his family, lovers, friends, and the wider world.

And it is the medicine women who birth these men.

Reflection Exercise: Cherishing Great Mother Meditation

Find a comfortable place where you can rest, such as a comfy chair or sofa, or recline in bed. Have a pen and paper nearby, as you may want to take notes on your experience after the meditation.

Gently close your eyes and soften your body into the place you rest. Relax your jaw, your cheeks, the muscles around your eyes, and breathe deeply into your body. Scan your body for any places that feel tight and constricted and breathe into them with Mother love. Imagine gold, pink, and fiery red-orange Mother love entering your heart and lungs. Place your hand on your sacred heart and invite it to open.

As you continue to breathe deep, slow breaths, begin to feel a soft hand on the back of your neck. Imagine this is the hand of the Great Mother—the strong, capable, and wise eternal Mother. She is looking at you with all the love of the eternal Mother for her precious child. Everything you do is perfect—you could never do anything wrong in her eyes. Allow her hand to gently press into those little dents underneath your skull, on the back of your neck. Imagine her hand pressing her love and strength into you. Notice what it feels like to be loved so unconditionally, to be touched by eternal love itself.

Notice now that your head is resting on her lap. Imagine her breathing under you, and with each inhale and exhale of hers, you rise and fall with the great Goddess—the source of life and creation herself. Take slow, long breaths with her as the two of you join in one oceanic breath. As you two rest and breathe life together, notice what she smells like. Earth? Sun? Moon? Dew? Flowers? Ocean and sky? Briefly look over her body and take in her gorgeous, stunning wings. What do you notice they are made of? Feathers? Metal? Wood or earth? Continue to stay with her, noticing her lap. Is it made of silk, velvet, moss, or something else?

As she holds you in her body, allow the Great Mother to use her other hand to gently massage your scalp and run her soft fingers through your hair. Feel her loving touch as she caresses you and cherishes you. Feel and receive her touch as she offers you her strength and nourishes you like a child. Notice how you feel as you allow creation and eternal love to hold you. Do you feel protected? Safe? Loved?

What else do you notice about Great Mother? Look at her sacred hands. What do you see? How about her hair? What else do you notice about her? Take your time with her. She is in no rush to leave her child; she cherishes her time with you.

Before you go, notice she is whispering something to you.

I love you. I want to know you. I see you. I hear you. I'm holding you. I'm not going anywhere.

Remember that you can always come home to her and let her nourish you with her strength, power, and love. All you have to do is call to her and she will come. She is a well of love, gracefully awaiting you.

Say your goodbyes for now knowing you can always see her again. Slowly open your eyes coming back to the room and begin to write about your experience.

JOURNALING PROMPTS

1. Write about your first impressions of the Great Mother and what it felt like to be held in the lap of eternal love.

2. What did you notice about her physicality, such as what she smelled like? What was her lap made of? How about her wings?

3. What else did you notice about her? Her hands? Her hair?

4. What was it like to hear her song: *I love you. I want to know you. I'm not going anywhere?*

5. Is there a man in your life who would benefit from this experience with cherishing Mother?

COMMON HURDLES
YOU MIGHT ENCOUNTER

- Projections of your own biological mother may come up, so try to remove images of your own mother and allow a new Great Mother to step forward.

- If you get agitated or stuck, try something relaxing—a bath, tea, dimmed lights—and try again. Don't force anything to happen; this is a receptive exercise.

- If you became too relaxed and fell asleep, don't worry, the Great Mother is very relaxing.

- You may get flooded with emotions: this is normal if you've been deficient in her love.

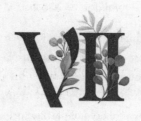

Saging into Mother

> She closed her eyes and imagined herself
> at the end of her days as deep
> in Crone as they come,
> And then she took a deep breath
> and felt the beauty inside
> Pulled it up and out, felt it rise,
> Then she looked in the mirror and sighed,
> "Gosh, I couldn't be more beautiful if I tried."

My Maiden-to-Mother work explores the radical truth that midlife is not, as our culture proposes, when a woman's power ends, but when it really begins. That power comes through an ancient initiation, a rite of passage out of the Maiden phase of reaching and becoming and into the Mother time of rooting and being.

Coming into the mature feminine is a woman's arrival. It is her bloom into the full moon phase of her life. This feminine life phase, the archetypal Mother, is a time of creative expression, sovereignty, maturity, inner power, and self-sourcing to the Great

Mother, who is within us all. If women were raised to focus on the love and purpose of inner beauty, instead of the emptiness and shallowness of outer beauty, by the time they were at midlife, they wouldn't feel invisible. They'd feel invincible.

Despite the oppressive hold of patriarchy on the lives of women for hundreds of years, there have been many, many women who understand the power of their blooming time. They are our ancestral Mothers, and for me, one of the most powerful is Georgia O'Keeffe, perhaps the most influential woman artist of all time.

My first experiences with Georgia were in the context of working on a documentary film about her lover, husband, creative partner, and the father of modern photography, Alfred Stieglitz. I was twenty years old and interning at a public arts TV station in New York. While this sounded very put-together, I was still neck-deep in unprocessed grief from my mother's death. I was a mess of a girl, lost in patriarchal programming, deeply attached to my weakness and fragility, utterly drowning in my addictions and deriving all my worth from my outward appearance. But the internship gave me an opportunity to latch onto something less superficial. Researching this most revered female modernist artist and admiring the raw black-and-white portraits that Stieglitz had made of her over decades, I identified a timeless role model of how women can follow their inner soul call and become who they were meant to be.

When Georgia O'Keeffe was in her midtwenties, she almost gave up her dream of becoming an artist. As a girl growing up on a Wisconsin farm at the turn of the twentieth century, when women had few professional options, her dream likely seemed preposterous to her social crowd. Yet she found a way to heed her soul call and was admitted to the most prestigious art schools in Chicago and New York City. With this education, she refined her vision, which wasn't to replicate the work of the top masters but to find ways for her canvas to be a personal expression of what she experienced in nature. Despite her promising start, she found herself back with her family again after her schooling, tending to her aging parents and their farm, all but giving up on her dream. While auditing an art course at the local university, she received some advice from the professor, who saw her great potential. He urged her to leave her family and pursue a teaching position in Amarillo, Texas. After years of doubting if any of her training and artistic vision would add up to more than vanity and self-delusion, she received this validation, which matched her own idea of her future. Her destination was an unlikely choice—the panhandle of Texas was a region of ranchers and churchgoers, often disrupted by the rowdy antics of gamblers and prostitutes. Yet she took the job and became the supervisor of drawing and penmanship for the town's schools. If she hadn't been pushed past her comfort zone to embrace her dream, she might never have come across this "big sky" country that inspired her most unique landscapes and still lives. "There is something wonderful," she wrote, "about the bigness and the lonelyness and the windyness of it all."[17]

Over the next several years, she continued to teach art in various southern and western locations. She knew that these places ignited feelings she had never felt before, things she was never taught, and that she had no choice but to try to express them in whatever way she could find. In her forties, she journeyed to the Southwest and fell in love with the dry desert of New Mexico. It was here that she made some of her most celebrated paintings of sagebrush plants and vistas. She never took a conventional path in her career but followed her passion wherever it led her.

Georgia O'Keeffe was a woman on fire with power and purpose. A woman who didn't give a damn about the patriarchy; who had shucked off society's ideas for how she should live; who had made the descent into herself and risen with the gold. She was a woman so on the edge of culture that she led it to new heights. This dissenter and creator dressed in simple black, wore no makeup, pulled her hair back, and painted her beautiful soul. She moved to the desert and gave herself over to spirit.

Her legendary life stood in stark contrast to mine. Georgia O'Keeffe did not care what men thought or how society viewed her. I looked to men for my worth and measured my confidence by how many social media followers I had. She did not care about whether she measured up to the culture's ideals of beauty. But what I looked like was all I knew of myself. While Georgia had liberating confidence, I had only shallow ideas of who I was, and my self-love rose and fell with how "hot" I felt. My psyche was entirely dependent upon what people thought of me. While I scrutinized all my creative work for possible flaws, Georgia famously said of her art: "I have already settled it for myself, so flattery and criticism go down the same drain, and I am quite free."[18]

I believe that for women who have lost themselves, or never knew who they were or why they are here, the spirit of Georgia O'Keeffe will find them and remind them. She found me again, nearly fifteen years after I first dove into her work, this time bringing me a very personal message.

Heading home from one of my retreats, I had stopped in an Albuquerque Hilton for the night. I felt like splurging, possibly to soothe my troubled soul. My room that night was a massive, climate-controlled white-and-gold-walled den in which I indulged in a room service order that could have easily served three. I remember thinking about the contradictory dynamics at play. With the money I made on a "wild woman" retreat, I was paying one of the richest families on Earth to pump carbon dioxide into the atmosphere and to support factory farming with my processed food feast, which mostly went to waste. Everything about my choices felt wrong, fraudulent, and misaligned. I was so far from who I wanted to be: a confident, authentic woman who lived true to her values. I just had the intentions, but not the actions, of a wild woman. My wounded Maiden was still so present in my life.

That is, until the first time that I ended up at Ghost Ranch in Abiquiu, New Mexico. That night at the luxurious Albuquerque Hilton, I dropped to my knees and asked Goddess for help. "Please show me the way," I said. And I received a simple soul reply: "Ghost Ranch."

I cocked my head, and I fumbled through my memory files. Ah yes! The place where Georgia did her most transcendent work. This is a wild desert canyon area bigger than the island of Manhattan, once called Rancho de las Brujas, or Ranch of the Witches, in Abiquiu, New Mexico.

I hadn't intended to visit there, but the morning after I heard that message, I was in my Jeep headed for the ranch. My first stop was in Santa Fe, at the Georgia O'Keeffe Museum. The black-and-white portraits Stieglitz had made of her were on exhibit, and she seemed to stare right at me through the camera lens, through the glass, saying: "Wake up! Claim your gifts and your power. I'll show you how."

I walked into a small theater playing a film about her, and I sat on a little bench in that dark room full of tourists. There she was, life-size in front of me on the projector screen, painting out in the desert. "It takes courage to be a painter," she said to the audience. "I always felt I walked on the edge of a knife. On this knife, I might fall off on either side, but I'd walk it again!

So what? What if you do fall off? I'd rather be doing something I really wanted to do."[19]

Hearing about the knife edge cut me open. I needed to have so many of my behaviors and defenses sliced away. I stood outside that museum, and I felt, finally, hot on the trail of me. I hadn't even really known I was looking for myself until I remembered Georgia. It was mid-March and a light snow started to fall, the white flakes fluttering down on the peach adobe buildings, releasing the smell of the surrounding pines. I had the feeling that I just might, if I kept going, find a life that was mine. I hadn't felt this way, ever, that I was on a treasure hunt and the treasure was me.

I needed to be in the place that Georgia dwelt, as close to the earth as possible. She had discovered Ghost Ranch in her prime Mother years, around age forty, and she eventually ended up buying seven secluded acres and a house on the property, painting its red and yellow mountain-scapes, dotted by junipers and piñon pines. I could barely wait to see it, this place that she had chosen to align with her greatest work.

When I arrived there, I felt that Ghost Ranch wasn't so much a first visit as a return. It was early spring, so it was still preseason. I had the place to myself, and the staff handed me a key to a lower-level cabin that looked like it hadn't been touched since the fifties. I laid on the musty green carpet next to an old heater and waited and prayed to hear more from my muse in the form of Georgia O'Keeffe. I waited a long time before she came. With my eyes closed, I saw her standing in her black smock, braced against the hot desert wind, her arms folded. She looked at me determinedly, challenging me with her fierce, erotic, strong confidence. "Whatever you need, you can find it here in nature," she told me.

I hiked out to a secluded canyon behind the main campus. It was so beautiful in the coming dusk, the air was peach-colored, and the canyons were glowing violet. The Great Chama Valley, where the Tewa people had lived for centuries, spread out before me. Winding through it, a river gleamed golden in the sunset light. Above, the Sangre de Cristo Mountains loomed, just as Georgia had painted them, with rust-red, pink, and ochre stone walls supporting the husks of battered cholla cactus and rabbitbrush. There, looking down at me from a canyon, still and quiet, massive and mesmerizingly beautiful, was a female deer. We locked eyes for a long, knowing communion. She was tawny and muscled, effortlessly graceful and intelligent. She bowed her head to me, and I did the same. Then she leaped into the brush, artfully navigating a path she knew, disappearing from my view. I stood there transfixed, grateful for this visitor, full of feminine power. She operated on instinct, reading the land, finding what she needed from nature's abundant gifts. Could I do the same?

While I had originally booked just one night at the ranch, I felt too deep into my slow, inspired, Mother energy that I ended up staying a week and lingering on my daily hikes through the canyons. I never saw the deer again, but I felt that Georgia stayed with me, guiding me on the trails she had walked and brought to life with her paintbrush. When I checked out, I said something to the effect of, "That was wild. I had no idea I'd stay so long." The woman at the desk took my keys and shrugged, "It happens to women like you all the time."

"Women like what?" I asked.

She paused for a moment. "Women who are looking for something . . . else."

I'd return to Ghost Ranch several times to lead Maiden-to-Mother retreats, offering to other women what I had received there from the spirits of the mountains and the creatures dwelling in them.

There is an arroyo in that canyon that I thought of as the River Styx, the river you must cross before you can rise again out of the underworld. I designed a ritual where the women would go to sit with their Maiden pain and allow these lessons to alchemize into wisdom, and then the Maiden pain would be given back to the water and the Mother wisdom would be kept, embodied as medicine.

In this ritual, women straddle the arroyo in a position that mimics how women used to give birth standing up, and how deer give birth, when their fawns are ready to emerge. They hold small Maiden dolls that they craft at the beginning of the retreat. They write their small Maiden traits all over the cloth dolls. Finding words like *envy, scarcity, smallness, jealousy*, and *fear*, they spell out emotions that arise from memories of something painful that happened to them when they were little. They hold these Maidens and then set fire to them, honor them as they burn, and bury their ashes in the desert sand, their hands digging and smoothing the ripples into small graves. As they wash their hands in the river, they announce the death of these traits and the rebirth of their cleansed souls.

One time while performing this ritual, one of my assistants wove a beautiful Mother crown from the roses that we had placed at the center of our retreat meeting circle for the week. After the burial and washing ritual, the women took turns crowning one another with it, anointing themselves as Queen Mothers.

I keep that crown on the rearview mirror of my truck now, and every day another petal falls from it and flutters down to the floor of the car. It helps me understand that women are like these roses, like the white ones that Georgia painted in glorious detail, close-up, with subtle color variations and an inner, glowing light. Our work is to bloom fully in our one life, because after the bloom comes the return to the earth. To bloom is to become more naked every day, to bear our true selves more and more. With every day, we lose another petal and draw closer to death.

Two other things die with the burial of the Maiden and the ascension of Mother. First goes her attachment to the fairy tale that she will be rescued from her life by anyone but herself. This is the death of fantasy: of crushes, un-acted-upon dreams, the idea that she will live forever, and that others are responsible for her happiness. These fantasies only serve to empower her and break her out of her glass princess case, to live, to act.

The second thing that dies is her external youth. Like petals falling from the shattered-open flower, her youthful looks that she once relied upon for external validation fall to the earth.

This passage is marked by her first wrinkles, the graying of her hair, the slight sagging of her skin. She is physically softening. This passage invites her to go within herself to redefine what beauty truly is. If beauty is not merely youthful looks, then what is it? In Mother, we know that beauty is self-reliance, creativity, intuition, resilience, grace, authenticity, compassion, imagination, service, humor, and vulnerability coupled with strength. She will reach down deep and allow these qualities to rise. Her beauty, from now on, will need no mirror or audience for validation.

Internal, eternal beauty will be what she loves in herself and what she is loved for. Her soul, her truth, and her gifts will be seen. She will be loved for who she is, not for what is fleeting about her. The death of the Maiden, if allowed with grace, gives birth to a new woman. While the Maiden carries burdens, the Mother carries gifts, and she is not looking for anyone to fill the gaps in her soul with missing pieces. She wants less, not more. Women in this transition into truth find they are moving through a portal—like the trees in winter, like a child from the womb to the world, she can only take herself. Nearly everything but the soul must be shed to pass into archetypal Mother. Houses, jobs, relationships, and not least, the patriarchal consciousness that structured the first act of her life, cannot come with her.

> To move from the
> Patriarchalized feminine to
> The mature feminine is to
> Move from
> Anxious to ancient.

One of the things I'm proudest of in my work is a reframe of feminine aging, or what I call saging (s-aging), which is the art of becoming sage, or wise. Aging is really a portal into power, a passage into wisdom, and it's a great privilege. This is a complete rewrite of the story we're fed about age, which is typically a story of loss that says: you lose your youthful looks, lose your sex appeal, and lose your ability to be seen and heard in a world where youth is preferred. But what do you gain? No one talks about that part, which is a grave omission because the truth is that we gain *so* much.

Older women in our culture suffer from these ideas of obsolescence. Our sexuality is derided, our physical aging process is grist for the comedian's mill, and many of us start internalizing this crone-bashing. Older women are depicted as wicked and self-aggrandizing—just think of the typical fairy tale's stepmother, mother-in-law, or witchy older women characters. The massive strengths of older women, such as taking care of people, guiding the emotions of their loved ones, and making peace among the immature, are mostly overlooked. When all you see around you are messages of decay, it's a fierce struggle not to respond to them with the negativity that reinforces the stereotype. Older women are caught in a patriarchal paradox.

Yet I boldly claim that saging into wise elderhood is a glorious process. As we soften externally, we strengthen internally. As we reject the culture that deems a woman's physicality her source of worth, we stop putting so much weight on our surfaces and claim a rising inner beauty. With that, our unrealized gifts rise, and they restore the healthy feminine to a world that is in danger of losing its nature. The saging wise woman keeps the vital connection to nature.

In order to find your inner wise woman, you must engage with the process of saging. You have to dance with it, you have to initiate through it—and if you do, the rewards are infinite. The antiaging industry would like to keep us trapped in this frenzied desire for something that's an illusion. Yet ill-usions make us ill. This idea of Forever 21, or staying in Maiden perpetually—or a frozen, plastic spring—is damaging. When we're obsessed with our outer appearance staying the same, our inside stays the same too. Your soul is meant to evolve and ripen and move through passages, and that doesn't happen if you are always focused on the outer facade, keeping it under glass in the museum of your youth.

As we recognize wrinkles and sags, creaks and changes, we recognize our mortality, and that is a gift. Our body is trying to show us we're mortal. How does the Mother respond? She's going to *live* an authentic life and not try to stay young forever. What a travesty it has been for the feminine to resist maturity over these past centuries.

There are benefits to others, too, when we sage. When we age in public, we provide safety and inspiration for other women as we claim our inner beauty. Not loving ourselves is harmful to other women because it causes us to compare ourselves to them. When you are comparing yourself to other women, there is no way you can be *for* them. If you measure yourself against them, you're naturally in conflict because you're seeing them as a threat or as greater-than or less-than. You must fully, radically accept yourself and come to understand your beauty as your soul's glory—an individual, unique force that doesn't need to be compared.

This happens when your Mother has taken good care of that insecure inner Maiden. Most women who grew up under patriarchy were subconsciously pitted against other women. We endured a propaganda campaign bent on creating in us an approval-seeking insecurity. When you've taken care of the Maiden and made her feel how special she is—when you're not comparing yourself—you are empowered. We need to understand the equality of women's beauty, in the same way that we can find every tree different, and none more beautiful than another. Once we start to recognize inner beauty, we can stop contrasting our traits with others'. We can start to feel rooted in that inner beauty and move to a soul-centered place of being in the world. When we don't see other women as competition, we can be on each other's team; we can root for each other. Only in that healthy, sturdy place of Mother can we serve in a way that will help other women.

When I saw myself through the patriarchal lens, I emphasized what was wrong instead of what was right. I focused on what was ugly and bad instead of beautiful and good about me. This is certainly an ingrained part of human psychology, derived from evolutionary threats. It's called negativity bias. All of us feel the sting of criticism and being shamed more than we feel the pleasure of being praised or appreciated so we can take quick action in dangerous situations. We tend to dwell on negative incidents, whether they are important in the big picture or not. Yet we have the power to reverse our evolved bias, especially in relation to what we say about our self-worth.

One of the practices I do with the women in my Maiden-to-Mother teachings is to have them tell themselves that they are each the most beautiful woman in the world. At first, the resistance is heavy. And then it softens as they practice in the mirror, again and again. I ask them to point out everything beautiful about themselves inside and out. Then the magic happens. When they see their own beauty, they can see other women's beauty. The comparison energy dies, and they begin celebrating themselves and each other. They go on to carry the practice outside our circle, remembering to silently tell any other woman they see: "You're the most beautiful woman in the world."

I also take them through a crone visualization in which they look into a mirror and look at themselves as they normally do. Even though we have been steeping in the ideas of saging, many will admit that their inner critic still starts announcing right away: "I look bad. I look old. My wrinkles are deepening, my maiden form is gone. I want to look young!" But then I have them put their hands over their eyes and begin imagining what they look like at age eighty-eight. I tell them to gaze generously and admiringly at their age spots, sags, wrinkles, and last remaining wisps of gray hair. When they can hold the vision of themselves as a Crone in their mind, I ask them to send their Crone compassion and love. When they remove their hands from their eyes, they see their current embodiment in Mother. They have new eyes for her, and more self-regard.

A final exercise asks them to imagine the inner beauty that stems from a deep motherwell inside that contains her resilience, grace, creativity, unconditional love, and grit to persevere. I ask them to visualize these qualities rising up the body and emanating out of her crown and surrounding her form in white light. Releasing their hands from their eyes, they see themselves and ask: How can I focus on how I act, rather than how I look? What is the most beautiful way I could *be* in this moment, calling upon my kindness, compassion, softness, and love?

I also encourage women to do whatever they want to make themselves feel in alignment with their inner beauty. For me, this meant giving up the color that symbolized Maiden to me: all shades of pink. In its place, I now choose red whenever I can. I claim rose red for my lips, to wear at the beach, to adorn my body when I want to feel like the beautiful, fully bloomed Mother I am. Other women I know have expressed their mature feminine through different fashions, jewelry, new beauty rituals, tattooing, piercing, and by wearing perfumes and oils that reflect the new woman they have birthed. As the author Anne Lamott wrote: "Joy is the best makeup. But a little lipstick is a close runner-up."[20] There's no shame in amplifying your inner beauty. Especially if we consider that Inanna was stripped of everything as she entered the underworld, as we all are. Now is our time to get dressed again. Or, like Inanna did, re-adorn as queen as she ascended.

What's exciting to see is how different and unique each woman's expression of her inner beauty is. There's no *Vogue*-approved, on-trend way to show up as Mother. What's most important is that we take the power of our appearance into our own hands, instead of imitating what the culture industry shows us we need to look like. This is not about sexual objectification, it is about sensuality, and enjoying being in our skin. The focus becomes how something *feels*, not how it looks.

Until you claim your own beauty, you won't feel safe around other women and other women won't be able to express themselves fully in your presence. You will depend on others and the world to reflect your attractiveness to you, but it is not anyone else's responsibility; it is yours. Continuously seeing beauty strengthens the Mother muscle. In Maiden, we gravitated toward receiving others' judgments in order to learn how we felt about the world. We were malleable to these external ideas and beliefs. Yet to come into maturity is to develop our own beliefs and radiate that beauty outward.

A Beauty Prayer for You

(Close your eyes and put your
hands over your face.)

Dear Goddess: help me to see
The True Beauty in me
Make me a woman
of Grace and Compassion and Resilience
Fill me with Self Love Peace and Sovereignty
Dose me with Grounded Serenity
give me the eyes to see my own and
others' deep and true beauty.

Reflection Exercise: Inner Queen Mother Meditation

Here you are, ready to cross into full-bodied and full-bloomed womanhood, into the archetype of Mother, the full moon and summer of your life. You must do this before it's too late and you die bitter and terrified with unlived dreams and unsaid things. We heal our Maiden not just to become Mother, but also for our Crone who comes in the fall and winter of our lives. At the gateway to the next world, Crone looks back at a life fully loved and lived and does not feel remorse and regret that she never got what she came for. We must also live fully before it's too late for the care and protection we offer the Earth. We are the Goddess's hands on the Earth. We must act now and become the woman of our dreams—our own powerful Goddess Mother. In this exercise, we first imagine her and then become her.

To begin, find a comfortable place where you can rest. You will want to have paper and a few art supplies such as markers, crayons, or colored pencils nearby. Take slow deep breaths, closing your eyes. Let the place where you are sitting or lying hold you. This is your time to practice being held. Whatever you rest upon connects to the Great Mother who longs to have her children return to her. Feel her pulsing and breathing in your body as your body becomes soft and receptive, opening as much as possible to the wisdom that awaits you.

As you slow your breath even more, start to imagine your most beloved place in nature—a place you feel safe, warm, and relaxed. This might be a beach, jungle, forest, desert, or another place near and dear to you. Let yourself fully arrive, taking in the serene and beautiful landscape. Notice how good it feels to be here. Imagine now seeing a cave in this beautiful place. This cave is safe, secluded, and part of sacred Earth herself.

Imagine that this cave that you see in this serene place *is* your own strong body. As you allow your body to become the cave, notice that there is an opening at the top of the cave. Allow yourself to approach the opening, remembering how safe you are. Slowly begin to enter the cave of your body. If you need help with entry, imagine entering the cave through your ear. Slowly take your time, and follow a spiral of stairs down, down, down, to the very bottom of the cave.

Notice the staircase is golden and decorated with gems and seashells. It is a staircase of ancient beauty, with thriving ferns, mushrooms, and moss growing in and around the railings and steps. Breathe slow breaths and continue to descend downward.

As you reach the bottom of the staircase, notice you are in a grand room. You realize immediately that this is the room of the Mother you've longed for. The energy is joyful, cherishing, creative, brave, powerful, present, unconditionally loving, wise, and peaceful. This is the mood of the Great Goddess, and you remember it from long ago. Continue to take deep breaths, hear your heartbeat, and relish these feelings of the Great Mother as you remove any and all blockages that do not allow you to unite with her energy.

As you begin to explore the room, you see a large, ornamented throne. Notice the details and materials it is made from.

It could be metal, or wood, bronze, gold, moss, or stone. There might be carvings or drawings on it. Now, imagine a powerful woman sitting on the throne. She is a glorious queen at her peak, in her fullest. She embodies all the attributes of your cherishing and most healthy Mother. Invite yourself to know that this is *your* inner Queen, *your* inner Mother, and she lives right here inside your great room.

As you come closer to her, notice how happy she is to see you. She is welcoming you and waving for you to come closer. She is absolutely delighted that you are here, and she wants you to take your time getting to know her.

As you approach her, begin to notice her feet, toes, and legs. Observe what she has on her feet or if they are bare. Are her toes connected to the earth? Is she wearing velvet or silk slippers? How about any jewelry at her ankles or toes? What else do you notice about this part of her?

Now begin to take in the whole of her. Notice what her body looks like and what she is wearing. What is the fabric she has on her body? Is she wearing long sleeves? A shawl? A dress or skirt? A robe? What color are her clothes? Can you sense her favorite colors? (Mine wears a glorious red gown!)

What do you notice about her hands? How about her fingernails? Is she wearing any rings? How about her arms, what do they look like? And her belly, is it soft or hard? What's her hair like? Is it long and wild, or is it short or shaved? What is her skin like? Does she have any tattoos? Piercings? Jewelry?

Come even closer to her if you haven't already and look deeply into her eyes. What do you notice about her wise, loving gaze? How about her soft lips? Is she wearing a crown, is her head bare, or does she wear flowers? If she is wearing a crown, notice what the crown looks like. Is it wood, gold, or silver? How else does she adorn herself?

No matter what, you can trust this inner Mother. She loves you just as you are, and there is nothing you can do to make her stop loving you. You are a gift to her simply by being. She is ever so proud of you and grateful for you. You are her dream come true. This is the Mother you have always needed but maybe didn't have.

Take in her essence—her power, joy, peace, kindness, ease, serenity, sensuality, courage, presence, wisdom, and strength. What other qualities does she radiate? Stay with her as she continues to welcome your presence and as you continue to remember that this energy lives inside you, this is your inner Mother, your wild Mother, your wolf Mother, your cherishing Mother, living right here in your inner world. The more you open to her, the more she will fill you with her radiance. From this day forward, your Maiden never has to feel abandoned or unloved again.

Now think of a challenge or obstacle you're currently worried about. Begin to explain to her your troubles about this situation. Notice the way she looks at you with great care as you share with her. As she begins to respond to you about this challenge, listen to the way she speaks—the way she responds with the highest love as she offers healing words to your situation. Her wisdom is strong and rooted. She may say a lot, or she may have only a few words to share with you.

She is telling you word for word the answer to the question: *What would the Mother do?*

Begin to wrap up your conversation with her. Step closer to her and embrace her. Notice as you embrace her that she draws you in so close that you *become* her. You are this Mother in her throne room, and you can always access her at any moment on any day. She and you are one and the same, in this flesh and beating heart.

Know her as yourself, bring her into your bones, this Queen Mother.

When you are ready, begin to ascend back up that spiraling staircase as Mother, embodied. See and feel yourself move as the Mother moves: unhurried, graceful, and calm. When you exit the cave, exit as your inner Mother and take your time opening up your eyes, coming back to the room you are in.

CAPTURE YOUR INNER MOTHER

When we allow space for creativity, such as drawing, writing, painting, and dancing, we integrate our experience much more deeply. Don't skip over this step! Here are a few ideas:

Playfully paint or draw a picture of your inner Mother, using any colors, designs, words, or shapes that came to you in the meditation. (This is not the time to be perfectionistic about your art because the Mother does not judge or criticize.) Some ideas to incorporate here (take what calls you and leave the rest):

What does she look like?

What is she wearing?

What adornments or tattoos are on her body?

How does she carry herself?

What qualities would you use to describe her?

What does she sound like?

What did she have to tell you or show you or give you?

How will you begin to embody your inner Mother in your daily life?

Practice playfully moving, dancing, singing, or walking as Mother. Or, simply sit as your inner Mother on her throne. Allow your movements, postures, and voice to reflect her essence and free expression. Feel yourself *as* Mother as you move and breathe the way she would. When you finish, write about your experience and what came up for you.

Write a story about your inner Mother. Let your imagination run wild as if you're interviewing her and this is her short biography of who she is, how she shows up in the world, how she is in relationships, what her creativity is like, what she yearns for, how she goes about her daily life, etc.

JOURNAL PROMPTS

What stood out to you the most about your inner Mother?

What did you notice about her "external" features, such as her hair, nails, skin, arms, hands, and so forth? What adornments did she have on her body and throne? How might you incorporate these into your life to feel embodied as her?

What did you notice about "inner" features, such as her essence and energy? What qualities would you use to describe her?

What wisdom did she share with you about your challenge? How did she speak to you?

In what ways can you embody your inner Mother in your daily life? And how can you remember to ask the question: *What would the Mother do?*

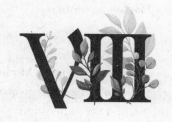

Mother Yourself, Mother the World

"It takes great courage to break with
one's past history and stand alone."

MARION WOODMAN[21]

On the journey from Maiden to Mother, there is a destination. It's a state of being—not of doing. One in which you always know how to return to Mother, what I also think of as getting back on your throne. When you were fully in Maiden, you didn't know how to do this, and perhaps you didn't even know that it was possible to become a woman in her full bloom.

It is my hope that this book and the exercises we have gone through have given you the tools to find your way through descent, rebirth, and bloom as Inanna did when she traveled down and back from the Underworld.

As we hold a circle for each other, we are healing a matrilineal line to return women to their power, to the collective remembrance of the pre-patriarchal, ancient feminine and their bodies. We are rewriting our story, becoming the authority, or *authors,* of our own lives. And in doing so, rewriting the story for the world. We are taking a left on the feminine path where our mothers only knew how to go right on the beaten path of their mothers before them. We are not betraying our Mothers to break with our patriarchalized matrilineal line, but rather, we are avenging our mothers and the Earth Mother.

This patriarchal pace
has proven deadly
for our bodies
and the body of Mother Earth.
For women's bodies and the body
of Mother Earth are one
And women's bodies and the body
of Mother Earth are done.
This patriarchal pace
leaves no space for women to be Goddesses.
And that's on patriarchal pur-
pose, for our Goddess,
and our connection to Mother Earth is our power.
And if we had more space to slow
down, to dream and to create,
The faster we'd birth
A new earth.
Because despite what we've been sold
What will fill that hole in your soul
Is to create a healthy new world
And not consume the poison of the old.

I told my story as an un-Mothered woman to show the effect of taking the Great Goddess from culture: you take the life out of the Mother and she becomes the Death Mother, raising submissive, fragile children who will never fight the system. Deeply Mothered beings, in contrast, have the confidence to take a stand for themselves and the world, and they feel the guidance and protection of the Mother always with them. Many modern women tend to go through endless breakdowns—like getting physically or mentally sick, or terrifyingly overwhelmed—to have a break through, or a break-out from the patriarchal abusive cycle. This abuse happens when you take the Great Mother—the source of life itself—out of a culture. All we see is death. When love is removed from the the culture, all we see is war. If soul is taken out of the culture, all we know is ego.

I think of Inanna as a lantern-leaver, as the Goddess who paved the rebirth path for us. She dissented and descended, leaving the upper culture for her descent to the dark feminine.

There is a way out.
And it is by going in.
Dissent and Descend to the Goddess within.

I think of leaving the abusive system of patriarchy as quite similar to leaving an abusive relationship. I didn't try to fight my shaman lover, I just had to get out. I had to leave to live. That reminds me of the story of one of my students, who kept trying to fight the system until it left her bruised and broken too, and eventually she found her way out.

Fernanda Parra, now a teacher of the Maiden-to-Mother work, found her way out of the patriarchy. A go-getter lawyer and mother,

Fernanda said that she had always believed that she knew how to do hard things, especially in an environment dominated by male achievement and the pressure to succeed in societally approved ways. "I thought that studying late into the night, writing difficult papers, and passing the bar exam were the hard things in life," she said. But then when it came to doing the work to heal her Maiden wounds, she got stuck. "I didn't know how to hold my personal pain, I hadn't really sat with discomfort."

Journeying deep inside to visit her Maiden showed her that she needed to expand her bandwidth to hold her emotions without turning them immediately into anger. "I learned to sit with my own rage and sadness and really truly feel, which transformed my being into more of the Mother," she said. By working to hold her difficult emotions and then express them, Fernanda was able to make huge changes in her life, transforming her career from the law to working with women and families, and leaving an expired partnership. "This work awakens the priestesses who are dormant in our lineage, they come back to guide us through." Every time she reaches deep inside now, she said she becomes more and more powerful.

It takes devotion and intention and ritual to hold ourselves in a Mother frequency that supports us in this way. It is a daily practice to re-member. To piece the shattered Goddess of the world and inside us back together through daily ritual. She can only come back through our bodies, and so daily we must embody her. We must continue to check in on our inner Maiden with Cherishing Mother love and support. We must remember our inner Mother and her power and strength and beauty. We must practice her way of responding to and creating her life, working our Mother muscle, until we get strong. We do so until the inner Mother dream is stronger than the outer patriarchal nightmare.

This is how we reject the outer nightmare and project the Great Mother dream.

The Mother *is* The Throne. She *is* the lap of humanity. The Maiden rests on her lap. The crone is at her back, whispering wise-woman wisdom in her ear. Your life can't work without you in the throne, as the throne. As the center, in your center.

Gather compassion for yourself if the mother who raised you didn't have this cherishing love for you—she never had it for herself. She had no model. You're the model. She had her own struggles and her own relationship with her mother, influenced by the restrictions of patriarchy. Death Mothers—controlling, neglectful, abusive mothers who keep us small and therefore sick—are patriarchalized mothers, blindly doing the bidding of patriarchy. All of this might have kept her from providing you with the kind of love you yearned for.

Through the process of this work I saw how my mother did her best with me and her life with the limited tools she had under patriarchy, and it also helped me realize that she did offer me many, many gifts. It took my own painful transition into Mother to recognize them. I often return to moments of my life with her, remembering the Mother wisdom she granted me

I, too, got sick during the writing of this book, just three years shy of the age at which she died. Before, I hadn't seen my mother as a peer, but she certainly would be now. I would be in her corner. I'd be rooting for her. Clapping. I'd be her clapper. I am now, and I always will be. I last knew my mother when she was in her forties, as I now am in mine. I could not see her clearly through my Mother Wound. But as it heals, I can see her far better. I can see a woman with a terminal illness, with two children and a crumbling marriage, trying her best with the limited tools she had under an oppressive culture. I have such deep empathy available for her now from deep within my own Mother Well.

For my mother's last vacation before she died, when she knew she had but months to live, she flew our family to California, a special spot from her past. She wanted to see Route 1 again, rent a Mustang, and hug the curves along the coast one last time. And that's what we did.

My mom had Eric Clapton's *Unplugged* playing in the CD player, and by the time we were on the highway, the sky was inky black, pierced with stars, and there were dozens of cars beginning to pile tightly behind us. And my mother went *so slow*.

The Gift of the Maiden Is Feeling as If She Has Forever
The Gift of the Mother Is Knowing She Does Not.

This was certainly the last time my mother would ever drive Route 1, or be in a convertible with the ocean breeze on her skin, or be on vacation with her girls, so she savored it. She felt and heard and smelled and breathed and saw every second of it. The horns blasted from behind and she turned up Clapton, while I hid my face in my hands. I was a sullen sixteen-year-old and slow was not a way I wanted to go. I begged, "Please speed up, Mom," but she held the wisdom of a terminal woman, that every moment is your last, so drink it like a fine wine. She was a guru for me at that moment. Her teaching was to choose the slow lane, to stay in it, to protect your peace, and teach others your pace. The last thing my mother said to me on her deathbed, in her doorway moment, was: "Find the joy."

The slow lane is its own ceremony. It's sensual, it's embodied, it's the path of the wise woman who heals with every touch and step. Women in Maiden usually come in fast, frantic, unable to commit, so anxiously concerned with "what if." What if I fail?

What if it's risky? What if the world ends? And so on. This creates a dynamic in which they are unable to be in the present. If you look to the full moon as Mother teacher, the only way to embody the Mother is to be present, to attune to the now. Women in Wounded Maiden wait for the good to come. The Mother is the good that comes. Women in Wounded Maiden navigate the world frantically attuned to what others are thinking. Women in Mother navigate the world deeply attuned to what they are feeling.

Similarly, after being diagnosed with uterine cancer, Marion Woodman chose the slow lane. She wrote in *Bone: Dying into Life* how she chose to prioritize joy in her remaining days. She canceled all of her appointments, made love to her husband, and walked naked in the rain. She took up dance as her body told her to. She kept listening to the guides of joy and ecstasy, the deep embodiment she was being guided into. After a long battle, one night on a Salsa dance floor she heard "We did it." The invitation of the sickness invited her that deeply into relationship with her body that she could now perceive changes in her body as clear as a bell. She was healed. Her cancer disappeared, through listening to her body's wisdom. She lived for another twenty-five full years, always ready to dance with and in the flames of life.

Like Marion Woodman, like Inanna, when in Mother we must live with the ever-presence of death, of others and ourselves. In Mother we hold the tension of no longer being young and not yet being old, but of our youth behind us and our death before us, like the full moon feeling the waning into the dark, like the fully bloomed rose feeling the pull of her petals back to the earth.

For Brandi, a dear friend of mine, merging into the slow lane and honoring the truth of her death so as to truly live came through an unexpected lesson in fragility. The mother of three girls, she lives off-grid with her husband in the mountains of Colorado. When Brandi found a lump in her breast, she decided she would heal it herself since she had no insurance or extra savings for medical treatment.

For the first time since becoming a mother fifteen years prior, she took time away for herself. Often, it is a reminder of death that impels us to live our lives more fully. Brandi immediately thought of a place in Hawaii where she'd spent some of her Maiden years. She traveled there for healing inspiration and waited to receive messages about her future path. Days passed, and nothing came. The quest felt fruitless, until the second to last day of her trip, when Brandi found herself sitting under a tree, feeling a bit desperate. She was in her last meditative prayers before she went home. Just then, a small, perfect, and pristine white egg fell from the tree above her, straight into Brandi's skirt. It was perfect, pretty, precious, fragile. She asked the egg: "Is this for me, may I take it home?"

In the warm, soothing voice of the Great Mother, the one Brandi had been waiting to hear, she heard, "Yes, it is for you. It will tell you what to do." Brandi felt grateful and relieved for this message from the Goddess. She wrapped the egg carefully in layers of clothing and packed it gently in her backpack for the trip home, which would involve two planes and a train. Brandi kept this egg, so tender and close, throughout the journey. She was unendingly protective, checking on it throughout the trip. Then she got home, knelt in front of her altar and opened the backpack.

The egg had shattered. There were wet, goopy shell shards all over. Shocked, Brandi welled up with tears.

"What does this mean?" she asked.

"What am I supposed to do?"

The same warm, strong voice returned:

"Let it all go, let it all fall apart.

Let yourself break.

Shatter.

Break Open.

Get Messy.

Die, before you die."

The egg is a symbol of fertility and new life. Yet, for the new life to come, the old one must perish.

"It felt like the breaking open of the universe," Brandi told me. "The big bang, my own little microcosmic explosion of life, screaming, with all the sacred muck."

The Goddess asked Brandi: Why are you holding "safe" all that is precious and holy; all the wild matter and sacred rage; all your variations of love; all the magic? Why are you keeping all of that inside of your vessel? Is it brewing and simmering? Resting? Waiting? It's cooked. It's ready. It can't stay in there anymore. This is a literal matter of life and death. Your "sacred container" is actually containing you. It is holding you back. The scream, the mess, the breakdown to break through will be your salvation.

"I remember a single moment of devastation when I realized the egg had broken," Brandi told me.

In that single moment of despair, she'd thought she'd lost the magic and the potential to heal herself. She'd thought the magic was held inside of this precious prize, this little prayer spell, this "nest egg." The next moment she was laughing. She understood that she *was* the egg, and *her power is not meant to be contained.*

Recently she told me about how well she is doing, and how she has brought herself back into healthy balance. "Sometimes

I find myself back inside the egg, and that's okay. There is compassion required in the surrender."

We must be gentle with ourselves. Rebirth is hard. It hurts. It gets messy. It is made of thresholds and initiations. Sacrifice is always required. But we know from nature what breaks out of the shell is new life.

Break. Open.

We need the women of this world to break open. We need the sacred, powerful feminine to stop self-containing. We need you wild and messy, full and untethered in the glory of the state of self-knowing Mother. We need you in your bloom, like the wild rose—beautifully imperfect. We need you like the full moon, and the howling wolf. Humanity has reached a now-or-never moment when it comes to our future existence and survival on the planet. Without women who stand as Mother to the wild within and without, we are all lost to the death trap of the patriarchal machinist and matricidal culture. We need you free and fighting for the sacred, with your wild, broken, shattered-open and turned-on hearts. Hearts in sacred, open bloom.

There is the hard bud around the Maiden to protect her innocence and her unformed self—she needs the armor to defend herself in the world.

She is still waxing and reaching up for her becoming.

Maiden is an individualized time. We are in the bud as if in the cage of ourselves looking for our life, our place in the world. We have not yet initiated into purpose and service. We have not yet surrendered to a life devoted to something greater than ourselves.

We find that life—that breathes like the ocean, endlessly giving and receiving—in Mother.

In Mother, there is no more reaching, only rooting and expanding.

But we have to break open. That is the crucial piece that we are not taught. They say, if you are listening, you can hear the flower screaming when it shutters open.

Stay with the ache, stay with the scream and dream of the new life until it breaks open. The bloomed rose teaches us that to bloom is to endlessly open, expanding to offer and reveal more and more of her petals, gifts, and beauty. More of her feminine essence. And the more the rose breaks open, the more beautiful, more powerful, and more nourishing it becomes for the feminine life in the wasteland.

When the women of the world come into full bloom, the world goes from wasteland to garden again.

The defiant beauty of the rose during the wasteland is a powerful teaching. Despite and because of the war-torn wasteland, she blooms. She rises through the cracks of the parched earth and, deeply rooted into the feminine well, opens and offers the nourishing feminine seeds to the world crying out for the Mother. The bloomed rose is a powerful symbol for a woman standing for love, for beauty, and for the feminine in the wasteland.

We cannot be hopeless. We must be the hope. We cannot wait for the good to come from elsewhere any longer. We must be the good that comes running. We cannot surrender to the nightmare. We must stand for the dream.

In this wasteland we cannot hide in the bud. We must bloom. To bloom is our feminine resistance to the toxic masculine nightmare. To bloom is to pollinate the world. To bloom is to keep an open heart through the storm, as guiding light to others.

But instead of blooming, maturing women have been cultured to dry up, to shrivel and be brittle, to break and disappear. We've found ourselves apologizing and self-shaming for the natural process of aging. We've been shamed for loudly living our lives past ageist cultural beauty standards that fetishize and center the Maiden, and desexualize and exile the Mother. We have shriveled and withered into the dust of the wasteland with this sick narrative.

Culturally, it is as if aging women are told to fade into invisibility. But on the feminine path, Nature is our teacher. And She teaches us—through the fruits on the vine and the flowers in bloom—that to mature is to become our most visible, beautiful, joyful, and alive. It is to ripen and radiate. It is to open your heart, no matter what.

In Nature, to mature is to open, to be plump and juicy and delicious and nourishing. To mature is to be ready, to be a *yes*, to sing alive with life itself. The artificial culture tells the maturing feminine to shut up and disappear.

Nature says that to mature is to become our loudest and liveliest. Nature is our teacher. Get up. Open up. Reveal your deepest self.

It is the most dangerous thing a woman can do, to keep herself in the bud and shut herself off from eros—the erotic life force that courses through her body. She is cut off from passion for life and she stops blooming. Her sacred feminine heart hardens and her magnificent flame dies. The world darkens ever more.

A woman's eros is her life energy—and without it she begins to wither from the vine and die. The autopilot sleepwalk begins, life is about what has to get done, never fun, never passion or play, no time for that, maybe some far off, ever distant day.

There's no adventure, no wonder, no pleasure, no mystery or ecstasy. It's all a chore and a bore. This can't be what a life is for.

Without life force the woman closes down and seals her heart off. The collective loses the gifts she was born to offer. Her life, without passion, is a slog of "shoulds."

But she has a deep choice right now to make within.

This choice may mean that she might have to betray everyone around her—to finally stop betraying herself. There is only one voice to listen to—and that is her own.

Only that voice knows how to break her open to her desires and tend her inner fire, only that voice will lead her to maturation and pollination.

It is up to the Mother to make what matters to her into matter. It is up to the Mother to birth the dreams of the new earth. It is up to the Mother to walk as Goddess to bring the Goddess back to Earth.

As a child, I remember how I kept waiting for my mother to be the Goddess. I, like so many women I work with, *remembered* the Goddess—moreover, I remembered a time when all women were the Goddesses—and yet couldn't find her in this lifetime. Desperately, I kept waiting to see the Goddess in my mother rise. My mother never became it, she never could, the Goddess was that deeply buried. Yes, I can now find some crumbles of Mother wisdom but not a life lived and celebrated in archetypal Mother. Like many, my mother was the patriarchalized feminine, which carried out the bidding of the patriarchy to subvert and sedate the feminine. (It feels important to say here, because of this Mother work, that I'm no longer mad *at* my mother, but *for* her, and all our mothers under the patriarchy.)

Subdued and made subservient, the girl never became the goddess, the Maiden never became the Mother. The death of the dream of seeing my mother in her power happened one fateful day when she came home from work. I remember so vividly, she got three steps in the door and collapsed onto the floor.

Back then, my parents were in the process of divorce and my mother had gotten a powerful new job. But in our misogynistic culture, there was gossip that she didn't earn it with her skills, but with her feminine wiles (the same accusation I'd endure some ten years later when I first began working at Rolling Stone). Even at thirteen, I knew what they were saying was not true, and she knew it, too.

But like so many patriarchalized women, the outer noise was louder than her inner voice. She got trapped in the room of "what others think" and never made it out. My mother must have felt utterly defeated to the lie to fall on the floor like that.

"I can't take it anymore, they're all talking about me," she said.

I couldn't stand to see her crushed under other people's opinions, projections, and lies. "Who cares, Mama?" I protested. "You know the truth. I know the truth."

"It doesn't matter. It doesn't matter what I know. They all believe it," my mother said.

The wounded maiden navigates the world frantically attuned to what others are thinking. Yet the healed mother navigates the world deeply attuned to what she is feeling.

I didn't want to look down at my mother—I wanted to look up at her.

"Get up, Mama," I said. "Get up."

She never did. Cancer started in her lungs soon after that and I had a mother that was always down, a mother that was always in bed.

I may have never seen my mother get up, but twenty-five years later I'd be on the floor myself, just feet away from my two-year-old daughter. I was crushed underneath the pace and devastation of the world, and I'd just had thousands of my hard-working single-mother dollars stolen from me. I felt hopeless, desperate for someone else's help. I was slumped in a corner watching her play, and I could feel my soul giving up as I wondered how we'd eat and pay rent.

"Get up, Mama. Get up," she kept saying.

She wanted to play, it was the middle of the day and I was slumped in a corner on the floor under the weight of it all. There was terror in her eyes looking down at such a fragile small mama, and I recognized it as my own. I remember how much I needed the Goddess in my own mother, an invincible warrior, the Wolf Mother, the Wild Mother.

"Get up, Mama. Get up."

I rose and I got up, and for the most part, I have stayed up—for my inner and outer Maiden.

As the Mother, as the woman at midlife who midwifed her own rebirth and has unlearned all she's been taught, I learned to tend to my inner cries, so I can tend to the outer cries of the burning world.

I got up, I am getting up each time I fall, for myself, for my daughter, for the world.

Get up, Mamas. Get up.

This book does not have a fairy-tale ending, and that is a deliberate choice. The story of Maiden to Mother doesn't end with me, or you, coming into Mother and then finding a dream partnership. I'd like to rewrite them all with the Princess saving herself and crowning herself Queen. As we all know, happily ever after is not the truth for most people. Instead, I offer the position of the Mother as a partnership with *yourself*.

When you can come into Mother, it can be your choice as to when you choose to renew or seek partnership with someone. The path of partnership is how some people become their whole, true selves. Some women I know choose to put only themselves at the center of their life. Or they understand there are seasons in their lives, and as seasonal beings there is a time for romantic love and a time to walk alone. In modern day, solo men are lauded as "bachelors." Solo women are derided as "spinsters." But in the ancient feminine, a woman unto herself, not married or belonging to another, was a type of moon priestess called "virgin." The archetype had nothing to do with sexual chastity and everything to do with being a strong and independent woman (*The Great Cosmic Mother*, pages 158-159). It is up to you to create your life, and being in Mother is the best way to prepare you for the next wave. And there will always be one. That's what's so wonderful about life. There's always a next wave coming. The question is: how will you respond to it? From the bud, closed and in fear, or from the bloom, open and in love?

The Mother knows: "What I fear, I will face."

Think of patriarchy as the paved path that has destroyed nature for convenience and speed and trampled over so many things in its quest to dominate. In Mother, you must leave the pavement and create your own natural path in the woods like a mystical deer who, by going a different way, symbolizes regeneration. Now it is your choice what direction you go in. You get to say what success and love look like for yourself.

At the beginning of my paved patriarchal path, I thought I had to chase a fire outside of me. I never learned the ancestral village ways of having my gifts seen and sung out of me. I never knew we all had a purpose. So I interviewed rock stars and movie stars, warming my cold hands over others' creative fires.

Often when people hear I once knew so many celebrities, they ask me, "Who was the nicest and who was the worst?"

You know who were "the worst"? The uninitiated rock stars or actors with one hit single or one big role.

The uninitiated ones, in their "Maiden time," who had never failed in public, who had never lost anything, who had never fallen down and had to get back up, who had never been brutalized by the critics and had to figure out who they are if everybody left, who were brand new and thought they knew everything, just like all of us in Maiden.

With the veterans, with the initiated artists, they showed humanity, humility, and the wisdom of maturity. They said: "I have lost. I have loved. I have had my heart broken. I have had dreams die. I have had the illusion of who I thought I was shatter a thousand times. I live low to the ground on my knees in deep gratitude for this life." Those are my people, those who have crossed into maturity and their humanity. That is true success and love for me.

There will be many times in the cyclical work of Mother when you may find yourself back in Wounded Maiden, or you will find yourself in the Underworld. There are many dragons on the way. We are not here to be successful on patriarchal terms. We are not here to be liked. We are here to serve. We are going to mess it up. We are going to stumble, slip, and fall, but that's okay. It happens to the best of us. It's not a question of whether you will wobble from your center and fall from your throne. It's a question of how self-lovingly and softly you'll return.

One of the most powerful things about maturity is that having survived so many initiations, you begin to carry deep confidence that you can make it through whatever you face.

Life happened to you in Maiden.

But life happens through you in Mother.

In Wounded Maiden, I couldn't handle anything. In Mother, I can handle it all. In Wounded Maiden, I was always asking if everything would be alright. In Mother, I rise every day to make it alright. In Mother, I face what I fear. I tend to what cries.

Like the goddess Inanna, you have sat in the throne as the priestess and the goddess of the Earth, you have aligned so deeply with the cycles of Mother Nature, you have watched her die every winter and come back to life every spring. The bigger your deaths, the bigger your births. You have watched the moon wax and shine so bright only to wane, fall into darkness, and disappear, but always return. You have survived a thousand fires, you have died a million deaths. The chances are high that you will survive this, too.

You have a very strong survival rate by midlife. You know where you're the help and where you need help. And you've learned to ask and to delegate as queen.

By now, you may have also gathered around you an inner council of mature feminine friends who would and could support you in this journey like Ninshubar did for Inanna. They say:

"I am not going anywhere.

I am going to stay here until you make it up.

I am not leaving your side.

I believe in you.

You are going to make it.

You were born for this."

Mature women need mature women. Mothers need Mothers. We know this. We attract each other. From a deeply rooted place, we root for one another. We are the clappers in each other's corners. We are each other's velvet laps.

For most of us who learn to embody the Mother, the wooded path will inaugurate us into the final stage of our lives: that of the healthy Crone. During the ancient era of Goddess celebration, a woman was understood to be a crone once her monthly menstruation ended, and a ceremony was held to welcome her into the final and most honored part of her life. Crones, the crowned ones, are the grandmothers of the Earth, whose wisdom is heeded by the community in times of transformation. They have deep knowledge from their life experience, their community with one another, and their sense of the preciousness of their remaining time alive.

Kamya O'Keeffe, a friend and Women's Rites of Passage guide, shares that Crones tend the thresholds between this world and the next, and as elders, they acknowledge the significant transitions in our lives. Historically, it was the elder women healers and midwives in a community who would be the ones present at the births and attend those at death. In every transition, the Crone listens for what is needing to be sung, acknowledges the pains and triumphs of the journey, sees and honors each initiate's gifts, and is also likely to make some mischief along the way. The Crone's ways of knowing come from Cherishing Mother but are now more closely aligned with the intangible, the sacred, and the spiritual as she inhabits the third waning stage in the cycles of our lives. By deepening her craft, the Crone sees that there is always more, more to let go of, more descent, more joy. She stands resolute in this season knowing by now, trusting by now in renewal and rebirth. Her very presence is a signal fire for those who will come after. By surviving the challenges and traumas of patriarchal culture, by continuing to live through personal and planetary grief and losses over decades of life, the Crone becomes the guide by showing youngers that she lived and learned to thrive, and you can, too. Through the truth of her aging, she has the power to restore the reality that life indeed ends, and that our days will not go on and on. In this the Crone deepens the Mother's reverence for life. Daily life evolves toward sacred ritual, and through her decay, the Crone nourishes life.

Marion Woodman came into her Crone stage because she birthed her soul legacy. She gave of her gifts and helped people all over the world understand the depth of the feminine unconscious. She became the woman she came here to be and did what she came here to do. She didn't just age and get older, she matured through a conscious process and become a wise elder. She could rest back into the wisdom of that elder-hood with a lot of laughter and good trouble. She could smile and let go instead of crying and holding on to a life that was not lived as her own.

At Woodman's time of death, in July 2018, rumor has it she said she had a wish—for every woman to have "a life of her own." This echoes the legend of Inanna, which shows us that a woman must ignore the warnings and judgments of others in order to go her own way. The times we are living in impart a special urgency to this message because we are in the midst of a planetary crisis with multiple dimensions. We don't have time to ignore internal messages calling for us to root and rise. We must do it now before it is too late.

For many, it may already be too late. Too late to stop the shootings, the brutality, the oppression of structural violence. Too late to save the planet from human devastation, and too late to stop destroying its diverse forms of life, too late to heal from the thousands of years of wounds that the patriarchy and systems of war and power have wrought. The wisdom of Mother can help us respond to these realities. We have to Mother up now, for the sake of the whole world. We must become the safety for ourselves, the rooted tree. Then we become the safety for the room, the community, the world.

How do you stay soft and strong in these burning and turning times where the pain can feel so immense and at times unbearable, where you close your heart off to survive, or you let it shatter open? When the world is getting harder, we get softer, when the world is getting hotter, we stay wet and bring the water. You break open, you shatter, and then you grow strong in the feeling of that unconditional love you hold. You *become* what you came here to be, and you do what you came here to do before it's too late. We need you to choose a different way, we need you to choose the path of Mother. We need you to consistently tune into the Mother frequency. Do not match the outer frequency. Choose an inner mother frequency. Every moment, we are blessed with choice. Come back to the River of Love when you get lost in the drama. Every time, choose the dharma of Mother Love over the drama.

So often the women I work with will arrive to my gatherings overwhelmed and nearly destroyed by this world and all of its very real sorrows. I understand why. They are often stuck spiraling down in the trap of fear and hopelessness that is so easy to fall into because of the realities of today. "What about the other people? What about all the ones who do not care? What if we can't do anything to help because the destruction is so immense? What if the world is bound to end? What if it's too late? What if, what if, what if?"

But the truth is that if we do nothing, then we lose everything. If we do not hold a golden vision for the healed, glowing-alive world we want to see, then it will never be. If we keep waiting for someone else to make it alright, it never will be. We are the good that's coming. If we succumb to the pain of this patriarchal nightmare, then it wins. We already know what happens if we let this world go un-mothered. When the Mother is taken out, the life is gone, and all you have left is death. The only choice now is to raise the frequency, become the Mothers, and decide the new future, before it's too late.

Patriarchal consciousness is a dying nightmare. Mother consciousness is a living dream. We must choose one. When the outer patriarchal nightmare is still strong, the inner Mother must be even stronger. Our work is to reject the nightmare and project the dream. That devotion to our peace, our joy, our pleasure, our creativity, the Goddess, and to the Earth has got to be stronger than the outer nightmare. We must root down into the ancient Mother Well, where all is deeply well, and from that place, offer our gifts to a dying world. From our deeply rooted and wide-open bloom, we must pollinate the polluted wasteland with the ancient feminine, with the essence of the Great Mother. In Mother, we can't look away from the crying Earth, just as a biological mother wouldn't look away from crying children.

Can we Mother the world? Can we tend to her cries? Can we lean in with love? Can we respond to her needs? Can we stand for the wild and sacred in her?

In Wounded Maiden, we may feel like the world owes us. In Mother, we know we owe the world. In Wounded Maiden we can buy the lie that someone else is coming to save us.

In Mother, we know we are the ones coming to save us.

When faced with so many challenges, the only choice we can make is to respond with deep presence and rich visions for something better. The only choice is to hold yourself in Mother, make yourself safe, make the room safe, make your community safe. Then make the world safe. This world needs you to live a life of your own. This world needs you to become a Mother to yourself and become a Mother to the world crying out for the Great Mother. This world needs you to become the bloomed rose in the wasteland, that fervent symbol of hope. The bloomed rose stands for the return of the feminine. She says that when the feminine returns to our bodies, she returns to the earth. And she is returning. Through you. Through your bloom. When all the women of the world bloom, the world goes from wasteland to garden again. Go ahead, do your part. Offer your heart at the world's starving altar. The world is drowning, and it's waiting on you. We're going to need all hearts on deck if we want to make it through. The world needs your medicine, woman. Leave the Patriarchy. Return to the wild. Leave the Father's house, as Woodman said. Return to the Mother's garden. Be the garden. Be the offering. Be the gift.

Get up, Mama. Get up.

Howl!

The Wolf Mother

Something is clawing from inside my bones.
It's the mad Mother, the wild
Mother, the wolf Mother.
We're taught so much, told to be the good mother,
but what about the Mother who sees and feels
a world dying around her, one in which her
baby—and all babies—won't be able to live.
The good mother will stay in her cage.
The wild Mother will rage.
What if growing up I hadn't been sent to
my room for my moods but been free
to express them in the living room
In a wild woman dance space
Crouching and growling
Crying and screaming
Until it left my body and met the stars
And didn't get forced down into
my body, becoming scars
Encouraged to howl it at the moon
And burn it in backyard bonfires
Dancing
dancing
dancing
Around that, too
Without our clothes, without our shoes.

Mother Yourself, Mother the World

Now we try to pill it or numb it away
but it doesn't go anywhere, it stays
in our bones and the earth
Poisoning us until the earth erupts
with pain and rage and
demands, demands, demands
its women leave their cage.
Open-hearted and sword in hand
fighting for a safer land.
I think I'm going to let her out.
I think I'm going to let her shout.
I think she's going to scream and howl
On one shoulder the jaguar
on the other the owl.
Scream with the fires
And cry with the floods
Let her rage boil in her blood
Cover her body with the good girl ashes
And roll around naked in the mud.
Act in beauty and courage and put down the wine.
The earth is crying, it's time it's time.
The wild Mother is writhing in my
hips, she's hissing through my lips.
My good girl has had her day,
She never knew how to live a
real, wild life, anyway.
My good little girl rests now, surrendering
to the wild Mother with a holy howl.

Reflection Exercise: Mother Rituals

Throughout this book, I have provided reflection exercises and practices for you to put the wisdom of the Mother into action in your life. By now, you may have a notebook brimming with your insights that you can reflect on to make sense of your journey from Maiden to Mother. Continuing your journaling in which you feel free to write poetry, compose prayers and spells, and write encouraging sayings to yourself, based on your daily or weekly observations of your inner Mother, will steady you in life's storms. My journal and I are tight, and without that writing practice I'm sure I would have fallen down further and more often. Putting my thoughts and inspirations out there helps me get up over and over again.

But it's also important to discover what *active* practice you may need in order to consistently bring yourself back into Mother. Designing a ritual that works for you takes time, and you may need to conduct several experimental sessions before you hit upon the one that brings you the most magic. Below are several suggestions for rituals that have worked for me and the women I have guided on their Maiden-to-Mother transitions. These might be done once, for a short time, or one particular ritual may become your daily go-to boost for embodying your inner wisdom.

I love this practice that comes from Adrianna Zaccardi, who is a guide for women based in London, England. She offers soul support for women through embodied movement and dance, helping to build intuition and soul alignment.

During the time she was in the Underworld, she told me that she started a sunrise practice in the middle of winter. "I started getting up at dawn and praying with the sunrise and receiving all of that natural beauty every day," she said. The practice helped her see differently, to always choose to perceive what beauty exists in the moment, which is "the frequency of the divine and the Goddess." She was more able to pick up on synchronicities and spiritual messages in her life as a result of this sunrise practice and commitment to beauty.

Is there a nature-inspired ritual that calls you? Many women I work with choose to

make powerful rites based on the cycle of
the moon or visits to nearby bodies of water.
On my first visit to Georgia O'Keeffe's
Ghost Ranch, I felt the wisdom of being
outside and communing with beings in the
environment, which helped me embody
Mother. How can you develop a practice
that allows you to witness and receive the
guidance of nature?

I've also experimented with several
different oracle practices that tap into my
unconscious and make my motivations
and dreams more apparent. Drawing runes,
consulting Tarot cards, and working with
other inspiration card sets give you a shortcut
to deeper understanding of your path.

You may also want to try the exercise
from chapter seven of telling yourself that
you are the most beautiful woman in the
world, which is always and forever your
truth. Draw your inner beauty up and out
of you, while envisioning yourself as a crone.
When you open your eyes, you will have a
renewed vision of yourself.

The ritual of creating a funeral for your
Maiden (chapter four), or crafting a doll and

writing all of your Maiden traits that you'd like to lay to rest (detailed in chapter six), can prove to be liberating. Take this doll out somewhere you can set fire to it, and then bury its ashes. As it burns, those traits go up in smoke, and in their place are your mature feminine gifts. To commemorate those, you can crown yourself with a flower wreath you slowly weave yourself, as you contemplate your unique Mother qualities.

These practices are often amplified by sitting in a circle with other women, creating a coven, and holding space for one another's feelings and transformative desires. Whatever way you design your rituals, keep in mind that the overarching purpose is to align with the values that you seek to embody in your Maiden-to-Mother journey. If you feel tension approaching this activity, know that fighting this resistance is part of the ritual, as you seek release into the woman you want to become.

Below are some more suggestions that women I have worked with have used to find their inner Mother, and I hope some of them will work for you, too.

MOTHER WATER

Have you ever connected with the water
you drink? Felt the nourishment, felt the
life-giving quality of water deeply? Here, I
would like to invite you to a daily practice
that can help you develop more of a
relationship with the water you drink and
your inner mother.

As witches, priestesses, medicine women,
and as goddesses, we can charge the water we
drink with the qualities of the inner Mother.
Ask yourself what qualities you needed
more of when you were little. Who is your
life asking you to be now? Maybe you seek
sensuality, freedom, playfulness, creativity,
deep presence, or unconditional love.

Close your eyes and charge your water by
holding it with the energy of one or some of
these qualities. What do you need from the
inner Mother in the embodiment you have
today? Hold the water container and imagine
that energy entering your water, into every
single molecule. You can also whisper or speak
them out loud, you can also sing to your water,
whatever feels right in that moment. Then
take a sip of your water with all the energy

you have charged it with. As you drink it throughout the day, your inner Mother will be constantly replenished with what you need.

Challenges and Obstacles on the Path

When you are traveling on the Maiden-to-Mother path, there are going to be impasses and blocks. You will have bad reactions and doubts, and you may encounter terrifying places, like those of old fairy tales. But this time, you are the knight. This is your life, this is your fight. It takes tremendous courage to be the woman who heals the matrilineal line by walking the ancient feminine way. Imagine yourself as that warrior woman, as that magician woman on the path to your throne and your sovereignty in the full moon of your life. The practices below will hold you during times of trouble.

Ghosts of the Old Story

Imagine that you get to a place and you start to feel your old patterns resurfacing. They are like the ghosts of the past around you, and you start to think that the painful thing that always happens is about to happen. Here you can stop and ask yourself:

"In this place, do I want to be a Maiden or do I want to be a Mother?"

Which one do I choose? Do I reaffirm the old story or do I create a new one? Probably, you know very well what your Wounded Maiden would do in this situation. But you may not know what your Mother would do, since you haven't embodied her consciousness before on this path.

Here I invite you to come into a practice, whether it's in your body, in prayer, or in nature. Wait until you hear that deeper, wiser, more loving voice surface. Wait and listen to her. That is the only voice you respond with to get past that impasse. Don't react with the Wounded Maiden constriction, which is the instinct rooted in your survival. You want to move from instinct to intuition. That is only possible with that new voice emerging from your depths, but it needs time and space to come into being. If you react from the Wounded Maiden, you are not giving Mother a chance. With a significant pause and some reflection, you can respond from Mother and change the story.

Dragon on My Path

There may be dragons on your path. If
you encounter one, you get really scared,
freeze, or get ready to flee. Your reaction to
this dragon, to this outer story or figure of
domination, is panic, trauma, and fear. When
the dragon breathes, its fire is presenting
you with a chance to heal your old story
as a medicine woman. If your reaction
to the outer story is bigger than what is
actually happening, something big must be
happening on the inside that wants to be
acknowledged and integrated. What is the
inner story here? Ask yourself: Why am I
reacting so powerfully? What do I need to
listen, witness, hold, and mother myself here?

Perhaps the dragon on the path is a
maiden wound the Mother is ready to tend.

And therefore it's as Rainer Marie Rilke
said in *Letters to a Young Poet*:

"Perhaps all the dragons in our lives are
princesses who are only waiting to see us
act, just once, with beauty and courage.
Perhaps everything that frightens us is, in
its deepest essence, something helpless that
wants our love."

MOON OVER THE WATER

When you come into your full bloom as
a woman in the summer of her life, you
will have responses that cause trouble. The
relationships you have been forming while
in Wounded Maiden may have difficulty
coexisting with your Mother. There is a
way we work with this particular reaction
in Mother. We know that the moon
influences the tides of the ocean on Earth.
If we imagine the moon as the Mother,
she never reacts to these changes. She
simply stays in her bright light, shining
and pulling with powerful gravity. She is a
force of nature, and nothing can steer her
off course.

The greatest gift of the mature feminine
is to first tend to ourselves, and then to
one another. We cannot give to others what
we cannot give to ourselves. How can I
ask you to love and accept me and live in
service to me when I have not been able to
live in service to myself? Mother says, "I
have all that I need, I came to give and live
a life of my own." The Wounded Maiden
feels like the world owes her, but Mother

knows that she owes the world. She must first show up for herself and listen to what she needs. To capture this mindset, there is a little practice I recommend in such times. When you find yourself saying:

"She is not listening to me." You can ask: "Am I listening to myself?" Anytime you dwell on these questions, you must turn it back on yourself.

He does not understand me. Do I understand myself?

She doesn't get me. Do I get me?

They don't care about me. Do I care about myself?

They are not seeing me. Do I see myself?

They don't love me. Do I love myself?

You are the witness to yourself. As soon as you can witness the Wounded Maiden and identify her needs, you can be her Mother, you can give her what she needs. Once that split happens, you can recognize her. To hear yourself is to heal yourself.

MOTHER MEDITATION: ROOTING DOWN INTO THE MOTHER WELL

When life's burdens are heavy on your shoulders, you can do a practice called rooting down into the Mother Well. I'd like to offer you an example of what that practice may look like. Read once and practice, so you can see how it feels for you. You may also record this or a version of this to play to yourself as you meditate.

Find a place to sit in a comfortable position and invite yourself into your body, into that place. Draw your attention to your natural breath, let your eyes choose if they want to be open or closed and begin to root down into the Mother Well.

Root down into the Mother Well. Let the Mother breathe for you. Let her take deep breaths, send that oxygen the way the trees send that oxygen through their leaves to you. Let everything breathe for you. Let everything hold what you are holding. Imagine the beautiful branches of Mother Oak reaching down to hold the burdens, the worries, the fears, the what-ifs you are holding. See what those things are, bundle them up lovingly, all those burdens. Pass them to the branches, to the arms of the Mother Oak. Let her hold and rock them for you, let her shush them to sleep. Your breath is the gift releasing each and every one of them with every exhale. Everything is breathing with you and for you. The Goddess does always come through for you every time. This time is not different. The help is all around, ask for it, be open for it. The Goddess knows your dream and she wants it for you, too. What she wants for you always comes through, let her guide you there. Goddess says: "I gave you this dream, you've finally said yes, let me take care of the rest."

Tuck your mind back to sleep, wake your heart. Harness all your Mother focus, send the Maiden distractions away, wake up, rise, reach out, and grow. Ask your heart what she knows. Ask her what she says. Ask her what she wants you to do at these crossroads. Ask her how she will navigate this path. And tell her that you are listening.

"I am listening to you, heart."

More ideas, support, and guidance are available for you at themotherspirit.com.

Recommended Reading

The following materials are recommended for women navigating this journey.

Blackie, Sharon. *If Women Rose Rooted: A Life-Changing Journey to Authenticity and Belonging*. London, UK: September Publishing, 2016.

Bloom, Ralph. *The Book of Runes: A Handbook for the Use of an Ancient Oracle: The Viking Runes,* 1982.

Brown, Michael. *The Presence Process*. Vancouver, BC: Namaste Publishing, 2005.

Estes, Clarissa Pinkola. *Warming the Stone Child,* 1990.

Estes, Clarissa Pinkola. *Women Who Run with the Wolves: Myths and Stories of the Wild Woman Archetype,* 1989.

hooks, bell. *Communion: The Female Search for Love*. New York: William Morrow Paperbacks, 2002.

Jenkinson, Stephen. *Come of Age: The Case for Elderhood in a Time of Trouble*. Berkeley, CA: North Atlantic Books, 2018.

Levine, Stephen. *A Year to Live: How to Live This Year as If It Were Your Last*. New York: Harmony Books, 1997.

Murdock, Marion. *The Heroine's Journey: Woman's Quest for Wholeness*. Boulder, CO: Shambhala Publications, 1990.

Recommended Reading

Perrera, Sylvia Brighton. *Descent to the Goddess: A Way of Initiation*. Scarborough, ON: Inner City Books, 1981.

Sjöö Monica, and Barbara Mor. *The Great Cosmic Mother: Rediscovering the Religion of the Earth*, 2012.

Sontag, Susan. "The Double Standard of Aging." In *The Other Within Us*, edited by Marilyn Pearsall. New York: Routledge, 1997.

Wolf, Naomi. *The Beauty Myth*. London, UK: Chatto & Windus, 1990.

Wolkstein, Diane. *Inanna Queen of Heaven and Earth*, 1993.

Woodman, Marion. *Leaving My Father's House: A Journey to Conscious Femininity*. Boulder, CO: Shambhala, 1992.

Woodman, Marion. *The Crown of Age*. Boulder, CO: Sounds True, 2002.

Acknowledgments

I want to thank Avalon, my precious brave kind joyful daughter who saved my life and raised me.

I want to thank dear Jaime Schwalb, who found me and knew I could do this and never let go of me—even when I was sure I couldn't go on! Thank you for believing in me.

I want to thank Jessica Kraft, the brilliant wild woman who midwifed this book with her whole Mother heart and crafty wise hands. Thank you for loving this work the way you do. Thank you for your patience with me. You're a true book witch doctor.

I want to thank my dear mother. I wish I could have known you better. I love you forever. This is for you. This is for us. I feel you. Let's walk forward together, hand in hand now. Patriarchy can't tear us apart anymore.

I want to thank my dear father. I am so grateful for our deep friendship and your gentle wise nature.

Thank you to my twin sister for our ever-evolving relationship and friendship.

I want to thank my dear beloved dog Gracie, who was my shepherd in every sense of the word and taught me unconditional love.

I want to thank Marion Woodman for existing!! For plumbing the depths of the sea of consciousness and bringing us back your rich nourishing dark minerals from below. For making us all feel less crazy and more seen and cherished.

I want to thank Mary Magdalene for her warm soft and strong passionate erotic love for Jesus and the Earth and holding me through all the dark nights and teaching me how to teach the women in circle. I love you.

I want to thank Goddess Freya for teaching me ferocity and passionate sensuality in Mother and Queen. For walking me through countless fires. I love you and your example of powerful brave sensual womanhood.

I want to thank Goddess Isis for . . . having me.

I want to thank Goddess Inanna for guiding me this entire time and offering me her teachings to teach and having faith in me as a bearer of them. They continually change my life. I love you.

Goddess Ereshkigal; for teaching me how to claim, hold, hear and be with my feelings. Thank you for holding our darkness for so long. It's time we took it back from you.

I want to thank the storytellers. I learned in this book process, I'm not a writer; I'm a storyteller. At first my ego balked and then my soul relaxed into my true skin.

I want to thank Perdita Finn and her Goddess brilliance and her spidery book midwifery.

Clarissa Pinkola Estes for culling the stories of *Women Who Run with the Wolves* together and championing feminine wisdom.

Georgia O'Keeffe for being a badass who came to me and slapped me back awake and pacing a ferocious fiery knife's edge path as an artist.

Maureen Murdock for writing *The Heroine's Journey*.

Amy Zintl for being my best friend and believing in me and this dream when it still only lived in me.

Acknowledgments

Lisa Russell, my original witch in white pants in the house by the sea.

Kamya O'Keeffe, at the Rites of Passage Institute in Byron Bay, and the mother to my Mother work and rites of passage work.

April Clark, my steadfast sweet and powerful director of coven communications.

Lynn Twist, cofounder of the Pachamama Alliance and the woman who healed my money wounds.

Molly Suggs, my womanager and steadfast support.

Bradley Haney, Bennett Blair, Annie Cattabriga, Laura Blakeman, Gizem Evcin, Allison, Boo, Atticus, Picnic, Sarah Jenks, Sarah Torinus, Nora Ephron, Britt Matkevich, Adrianna Zajonc, McKenzie Zaccardi, Dana Myers, Nancy Meyers, Eddie Vedder, Ghost Ranch, Martha's Vineyard, all the witches, wisewomen, and priestesses who walked before, everyone who touched this book in some form. Thank you Gizem for final Mother touches.

I want to thank all my Maiden-to-Mother students ever, all the women with the courage to walk this path—rather, their path. I want to thank my teacher trainers—right now I'm thinking of the Maiden Voyage and the fire we walked through together. Each of you is part of my body now. I want to thank my current and future teacher trainers for carrying this work out into the world and helping the women remember.

Thank you to our ancestors for these rituals and ceremonies that have lived on in winds whispers and our very bones and blood, as much still in the mycelium of the forest as it is in my cells.

Goddess bless you.

Healing to the people,

creatures, land, air, and sea,

Healing to the Mother within

you and me.

Endnotes

INTRODUCTION

1. Marion Woodman, *Coming Home to Myself: Reflections for Nurturing a Woman's Body and Soul* (Niagara, NY: Mango Media, 2020).

CHAPTER 1

2. Elizabeth Appell, Class Schedule, January 1979 (Orinda, CA: John F. Kennedy University, 1979).
3. Rainer M. Rilke, *Letters to a Young Poet*, trans. M. D. Herter Norton (New York: W. W. Norton & Company, 1934).

CHAPTER 2

4. Monica Sjöö and Barbara Mor, *The Great Cosmic Mother: Rediscovering the Religion of the Earth* (San Francisco, CA: HarperOne, 2012).
5. Joseph Campbell, *A Joseph Campbell Companion: Reflections on the Art of Living*, ed. Diane K. Osbon (New York: Harper Perennial, 1998).

CHAPTER 3

6. Carl G. Jung, "Instinct and the Unconscious" in *Collected Works of C. G. Jung, Volume 8: Structure &*

Dynamics of the Psyche, ed. Gerhard Adler and R. F. C. Hull (Princeton: Princeton University Press, 2014), 129–138. doi.org/10.1515/9781400850952.129.

7. Stephen Jenkinson, *Orphan Wisdom*, orphanwisdom.com/.

CHAPTER 4

8. Alanis Morissette, *Feast on Scraps*, Maverick, Warner Bros., Warner Music Vision, 2002, compact disc.

9. Maureen Murdock, *The Heroine's Journey* (Boston, MA: Shambhala, 2020).

10. Starhawk, *The Spiral Dance* (New York: Harper & Row, 1979).

CHAPTER 5

11. Carl G. Jung, *Synchronicity: An Acausal Connecting Principle* (Princeton: Princeton University Press, 2012), 44.

12. Gary Osborn, "Gate of God: Ishtar's Descent into the Underworld," 2012, garyosborn.moonfruit.com/ishtars-descent/4572753514.

13. Amanda Yates Garcia, *Initiated: Memoir of a Witch* (New York: Grand Central Publishing, 2021).

CHAPTER 6

14. Lawrence Greenwood (aka Whitley), "More than Life," *The Submarine*, Dew Process Records, 2007.

15. Adrienne Rich, *Of Woman Born: Motherhood as Experience and Institution* (New York: W. W. Norton & Company, 2021).

16. bell hooks, *Understanding Patriarchy* (Louisville, KY: Louisville Anarchist Federation Federation, 2010).

CHAPTER 7

17. Georgia O'Keeffe, *Lovingly, Georgia: The Complete Correspondence of Georgia O'Keeffe and Anita Pollitzer* (New York: Simon & Schuster, 1990).

18. Georgia O'Keeffe, *Georgia O'Keeffe* (New York: Viking Press, 1976).

19. Karin Haanappel, "Georgia O'Keeffe: A Life in Art," 2013, YouTube video, youtube.com/watch?v=NV1w0IK_sdA.

20. Anne Lamott, *Grace (Eventually): Thoughts on Faith* (New York: Penguin, 2008).

CHAPTER 8

21. Marion Woodman, *Addiction to Perfection: The Still Unravished Bride: A Psychological Study* (Brantford, ON: W. Ross MacDonald School Resource Services Library, 2009).

About the Author

Sarah Durham Wilson is a women's rites of passage leader and writer. She is the founder of The MotherSpirit, which focuses on archetypal Mother work and resurrecting the rite of passage from Maiden to Mother. She has taught courses and led retreats for hundreds of women over the past decade and works with private clients. She previously worked as an arts and music writer in New York City, writing for *Rolling Stone*, *GQ*, *Vanity Fair*, and *Interview* magazines and VH1. In 2010, she began to write under the pen name DOITGIRL, which provided inspiration for women waking to the path of the witch and priestess. She lives on Martha's Vineyard with her daughter Avalon and black cat familiar, Odin. themotherspirit.com

About Sounds True

Sounds True is a multimedia publisher whose mission is to inspire and support personal transformation and spiritual awakening. Founded in 1985 and located in Boulder, Colorado, we work with many of the leading spiritual teachers, thinkers, healers, and visionary artists of our time. We strive with every title to preserve the essential "living wisdom" of the author or artist. It is our goal to create products that not only provide information to a reader or listener but also embody the quality of a wisdom transmission.

For those seeking genuine transformation, Sounds True is your trusted partner. At SoundsTrue.com you will find a wealth of free resources to support your journey, including exclusive weekly audio interviews, free downloads, interactive learning tools, and other special savings on all our titles.

To learn more, please visit SoundsTrue.com/freegifts or call us toll-free at 800.333.9185.

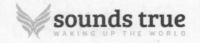